# EXAMINING CHALLENGES AND POSSIBLE STRATEGIES TO STRENGTHEN U.S. HEALTH SECURITY

## PROCEEDINGS OF A WORKSHOP

Anna Nicholson, Lisa Brown, and Justin Snair, *Rapporteurs*

Forum on Medical and Public Health Preparedness for Disasters and Emergencies

Board on Health Sciences Policy

Health and Medicine Division

*The National Academies of*
SCIENCES · ENGINEERING · MEDICINE



THE NATIONAL ACADEMIES PRESS
*Washington, DC*
**www.nap.edu**

THE NATIONAL ACADEMIES PRESS 500 Fifth Street, NW Washington, DC 20001

This project was jointly supported by contracts between the National Academy of Sciences and the American College of Emergency Physicians; American Hospital Association; American Red Cross; Association of Public Health Laboratories; Association of State and Territorial Health Officials; Child Care Aware of America; Council of State and Territorial Epidemiologists; East West Protection; Emergency Nurses Association; GlaxoSmithKline; Healthcare Ready; Infectious Diseases Society of America; Meridian Medical Technologies; National Association of Chain Drug Stores; National Association of County & City Health Officials; National Association of Emergency Medical Technicians; Robert Wood Johnson Foundation (Contract No. ID#: 73289); Seqirus; Trauma Center Association of America, U.S. Centers for Disease Control and Prevention (Contract No. 200-2011-38807, TO #54); U.S. Department of Defense (Contract No. HHSP233201400020B/HHSP23337014); U.S. Department of Defense, Uniformed Services University of the Health Sciences (Contract No. HU0001-16-1-0022); U.S. Department of Health and Human Services' Administration for Children and Families (Contract No. HHSP233201400153P); U.S. Department of Health and Human Services' National Institutes of Health: National Institute of Allergy and Infectious Diseases, National Institute of Environmental Sciences, and National Library of Medicine (Contract No. HHSN26300084); U.S. Department of Health and Human Services' Office of the Assistant Secretary for Preparedness and Response (Contract No. HHSO100201550005A); U.S. Department of Health and Human Services' U.S. Food and Drug Administration (Contract No. 1R13FD005495-01); U.S. Department of Homeland Security, Office of Health Affairs (Contract No. HSHQDC-15-C-00079); and U.S. Department of Transportation and the National Highway Traffic Safety Administration (Contract No. DTNH22-14-H-00468). Any opinions, findings, conclusions, or recommendations expressed in this publication do not necessarily reflect the views of any organization or agency that provided support for the project.

International Standard Book Number-13: 978-0-309-46375-1
International Standard Book Number-10: 0-309-46375-0
Digital Object Identifier: https://doi.org/10.17226/24856

Additional copies of this publication are available for sale from the National Academies Press, 500 Fifth Street, NW, Keck 360, Washington, DC 20001; (800) 624-6242 or (202) 334-3313; http://www.nap.edu.



Printed in the United States of America

Suggested citation: National Academies of Sciences, Engineering, and Medicine. 2018. *Examining challenges and possible strategies to strengthen U.S. health security: Proceedings of a workshop.* Washington, DC: The National Academies Press. doi: https://doi.org/10.17226/24856.

*The National Academies of*

# SCIENCES • ENGINEERING • MEDICINE

The **National Academy of Sciences** was established in 1863 by an Act of Congress, signed by President Lincoln, as a private, nongovernmental institution to advise the nation on issues related to science and technology. Members are elected by their peers for outstanding contributions to research. Dr. Marcia McNutt is president.

The **National Academy of Engineering** was established in 1964 under the charter of the National Academy of Sciences to bring the practices of engineering to advising the nation. Members are elected by their peers for extraordinary contributions to engineering. Dr. C. D. Mote, Jr., is president.

The **National Academy of Medicine** (formerly the Institute of Medicine) was established in 1970 under the charter of the National Academy of Sciences to advise the nation on medical and health issues. Members are elected by their peers for distinguished contributions to medicine and health. Dr. Victor J. Dzau is president.

The three Academies work together as the **National Academies of Sciences, Engineering, and Medicine** to provide independent, objective analysis and advice to the nation and conduct other activities to solve complex problems and inform public policy decisions. The National Academies also encourage education and research, recognize outstanding contributions to knowledge, and increase public understanding in matters of science, engineering, and medicine.

Learn more about the National Academies of Sciences, Engineering, and Medicine at **www.nationalacademies.org**.

*The National Academies of*

SCIENCES · ENGINEERING · MEDICINE

## PLANNING COMMITTEE ON OPPORTUNITIES FOR THE FUTURE OF HEALTH CARE AND PUBLIC HEALTH PREPAREDNESS, RESPONSE, AND RECOVERY[1]

**THOMAS V. INGLESBY** (*Chair*), Director, Center for Health Security, Johns Hopkins Bloomberg School of Public Health
**DAVID M. ABRAMSON,** Professor, College of Global Public Health, New York University
**MARY CASEY-LOCKYER,** Senior Associate, Disaster Health Program Development, American Red Cross
**BROOKE COURTNEY,** Senior Regulatory Counsel, Office of Counterterrorism and Emerging Threats, U.S. Food and Drug Administration, U.S. Department of Health and Human Services
**JON R. KROHMER,** Director, National Highway Traffic Safety Administration, U.S. Department of Transportation
**EMILY LORD,** Executive Director, Healthcare Ready
**SUZET M. McKINNEY,** Executive Director, Illinois Medical District Commission
**JOHN OSBORN,** Operations Manager, Assistant Professor, Health Care Systems Engineering, Department of Surgery, Mayo Clinic College of Medicine
**TARA O'TOOLE,** Senior Fellow, Executive Vice President, In-Q-Tel
**RAJIV RAMNATH,** Director, National Science Foundation
**TIMOTHY L. SELLNOW,** Professor, University of Central Florida
**W. CRAIG VANDERWAGEN,** Co-Founder and Director, East West Protection, LLC
**SANDRA WHITEHEAD,** Manager, Program and Partnership Development, National Environmental Health Association
**LAURA WOLF,** Chief, Critical Infrastructure Protection Branch, U.S. Department of Health and Human Services

*Health and Medicine Division Staff*

**JUSTIN SNAIR,** Senior Program Officer (until September 2017)
**CLAIRE GIAMMARIA,** Associate Program Officer
**ALEXA EDMIER,** Research Assistant
**ALEX REPACE,** Senior Program Assistant
**ANDREW M. POPE,** Director, Board on Health Sciences Policy

[1] The National Academies of Sciences, Engineering, and Medicine's planning committees are solely responsible for organizing the workshop, identifying topics, and choosing speakers. The responsibility for the published Proceedings of a Workshop rests with the workshop rapporteurs and the institution.

*Consultants*

**ANNA NICHOLSON,** Doxastic Communications
**LAURA RUNNELS,** LAR Consulting

## FORUM ON MEDICAL AND PUBLIC HEALTH PREPAREDNESS FOR DISASTERS AND EMERGENCIES[1]

**DAN HANFLING** (*Co-Chair*), Clinical Professor, Department of Emergency Medicine; Contributing Scholar, Center for Health Security, Johns Hopkins Bloomberg School of Public Health

**SUZET M. McKINNEY** (*Co-Chair*), Executive Director, Illinois Medical District Commission

**ROY L. ALSON,** Associate Professor, Emergency Medicine, Wake Forest School of Medicine; Representative, American College of Emergency Physicians

**STACEY J. ARNESEN,** Branch Chief, Disaster Information Management Research Center, National Library of Medicine, National Institutes of Health, U.S. Department of Health and Human Services

**PAMELA BLACKWELL,** Director, Center for Emergency Preparedness and Response, Cobb/Douglas Boards of Health; Representative, National Association of County & City Health Officials

**ERIC C. BLANK,** Senior Director, Public Health Programs and Systems, Association of Public Health Laboratories

**JAMES S. BLUMENSTOCK,** Chief, Health Security, Association of State and Territorial Health Officials (since October 2017)

**KATHRYN BRINSFIELD,** Assistant Secretary of Health Affairs and Chief Medical Officer, Office of Health Affairs, U.S. Department of Homeland Security (until January 2017)

**MARY CASEY-LOCKYER,** Senior Associate, Disaster Health Program Development, American Red Cross (since May 2017)

**BROOKE COURTNEY,** Senior Regulatory Counsel, Office of Counterterrorism and Emerging Threats, U.S. Food and Drug Administration, U.S. Department of Health and Human Services

**RICHARD N. DANILA,** Epidemiology Program Manager, Deputy State Epidemiologist, Minnesota Department of Health; Representative, Council for State and Territorial Epidemiologists (until October 2017)

**DAVID EISENMAN,** Director, Center for Public Health and Disasters, David Geffen School of Medicine and the Fielding School of Public Health, University of California, Los Angeles (since August 2017)

**BRUCE EVANS,** Fire Chief, Upper Pine River Fire Protection District; Representative, National Association of Emergency Medical Technicians

---

[1] The National Academies of Sciences, Engineering, and Medicine's forums do not issue, review, or approve individual documents. The responsibility for the published Proceedings of a Workshop rests with the workshop rapporteurs and the institution.

**LARRY (DAVE) FLUTY,** Acting Assistant Secretary, Office of Health Affairs, U.S. Department of Health and Human Services (since January 2017)

**ROBERTO GARZA,** Acting Deputy Director, Office of Public Health Preparedness and Response, Administration of Children and Families, U.S. Department of Health and Human Services (since May 2017)

**JOHN L. HICK,** Associate Medical Director, Emergency Medical Services; Medical Director, Emergency Medicine, Hennepin County Medical Center

**ROBERT KADLEC,** Office of Assistant Secretary for Preparedness and Response, U.S. Department of Health and Human Services (since October 2017)

**CLAUDIA M. KELLY,** Senior Director, Value Access and Policy, Seqirus

**THOMAS KIRSCH,** Director, National Center for Disaster Medicine Public Health; Professor, Military and Emergency Medicine, Uniformed Services University of the Health Sciences, U.S. Department of Defense

**GEORGE W. KORCH,** Acting Assistant Secretary for Preparedness and Response, Office of the Assistant Secretary for Preparedness and Response, U.S. Department of Health and Human Services (until October 2017)

**MICHAEL G. KURILLA,** Director, Office of Biodefense Research Affairs; Associate Director, BioDefense Product Development, National Institute of Allergy and Infectious Diseases, National Institutes of Health, U.S. Department of Health and Human Services

**DREW E. LEWIS,** Medical Lead, Clinical Research and Medical Operations, Meridian Medical Technologies (since February 2017)

**EMILY LORD,** Executive Director, Healthcare Ready (until May 2017)

**NICOLETTE A. LOUISSAINT,** Director, Programming, Healthcare Ready (since June 2017)

**NICOLE LURIE,** Assistant Secretary for Preparedness and Response, Office of the Assistant Secretary for Preparedness and Response, U.S. Department of Health and Human Services (until January 2017)

**FREDA GAIL LYON,** Vice President, Emergency Services, WellStar Health System; Representative, Emergency Nurses Association

**AUBREY K. MILLER,** Captain, U.S. Public Health Service; Senior Medical Advisor, Office of the Director, National Institute of Environmental Health Sciences, National Institutes of Health, U.S. Department of Health and Human Services

**JOHN OSBORN,** Operations Manager, Assistant Professor, Health Care Systems Engineering, Department of Surgery, Mayo Clinic College of Medicine

**TARA O'TOOLE,** Senior Fellow, Executive Vice President, In-Q-Tel

**ANDREW T. PAVIA,** Professor, Division Pediatric Infectious Diseases, University of Utah; Representative, Infectious Diseases Society of America

**JENNIFER PIPA,** Senior Director of Recovery Operations, American Red Cross (until April 2017)

**ALONZO PLOUGH,** Vice President, Research-Evaluation-Learning; Chief Science Officer, Robert Wood Johnson Foundation

**TERRY RAUCH,** Program Director, Defense Medicine Research and Development, Office of the Assistant Secretary of Defense for Health Affairs, U.S. Department of Defense (since June 2017)

**STEPHEN C. REDD,** Director, Office of Public Health Preparedness and Response, U.S. Centers for Disease Control and Prevention, U.S. Department of Health and Human Services

**MARY J. RILEY,** Director, Office of Human Services Emergency Preparedness Response; Captain, U.S. Public Health Service, Administration for Children and Families, U.S. Department of Health and Human Services (until February 2017)

**ANDREW R. ROSZAK,** Senior Director of Emergency Preparedness, Child Care Aware of America (until January 2017)

**SARA E. ROSZAK,** Director, Research, National Association of Chain Drug Stores

**ROSLYNE SCHULMAN,** Director, Policy Development, American Hospital Association

**RICHARD A. SERINO,** Distinguished Visiting Fellow, National Preparedness Leadership Initiative; Senior Advisor, Harvard University School of Public Health

**ALAN SINISCALCHI,** Surveillance Coordinator for Influenza, Bioterrorism, and Public Health, State of Connecticut Department of Public Health; Representative, Council of State and Territorial Epidemiologists

**MONCEF M. SLAOUI,** Chairman, Global Vaccines, GlaxoSmithKline (until May 2017)

**DAVID J. SMITH,** Deputy Assistant Secretary of Defense, Health Readiness, Policy and Oversight, U.S. Department of Defense (until May 2017)

**W. CRAIG VANDERWAGEN,** Co-Founder and Director, East West Protection, LLC

**JENNIFER WARD,** President, Trauma Center Association of America

**COLE WEEKS,** Deputy Director, Office of Human Services Emergency Preparedness and Response, Administration for Children and Families, U.S. Department of Health and Human Services (until May 2017)

**JOHN WIESMAN,** Secretary of Health, Office of the Secretary, Washington State Department of Health; Representative, Association for State and Territorial Health Officials

**GAMUNU WIJETUNGE,** EMS Specialist, Office of Emergency Medical Services, National Highway Traffic Safety Administration, U.S. Department of Transportation

**MATTHEW K. WYNIA,** Director, Center for Bioethics and Humanities, University of Colorado Denver

*Health and Medicine Division Staff*

**JUSTIN SNAIR,** Senior Program Officer (until September 2017)
**LISA BROWN,** Program Officer
**MORGAN BONAME,** Associate Program Officer (until January 2018)
**CLAIRE GIAMMARIA,** Associate Program Officer (from February 2017)
**JOANNA ROBERTS,** Research Associate (until August 2017)
**ALEXA EDMIER,** Research Assistant (until November 2017)
**ALEX REPACE,** Senior Program Assistant
**ANDREW M. POPE,** Director, Board on Health Sciences Policy

# Reviewers

This Proceedings of a Workshop was reviewed in draft form by individuals chosen for their diverse perspectives and technical expertise. The purpose of this independent review is to provide candid and critical comments that will assist the National Academies of Sciences, Engineering, and Medicine in making each published proceedings as sound as possible and to ensure that it meets the institutional standards for quality, objectivity, evidence, and responsiveness to the charge. The review comments and draft manuscript remain confidential to protect the integrity of the process.

We thank the following individuals for their review of this proceedings:

**KATIE SCHEMM DWYER,** National Association of County & City Health Officials
**DOUG HALLEY,** CrossTown Connect
**PUNEET KHAN,** The Cadmus Group LLC
**LEESA LIN,** Harvard T.H. Chan School of Public Health
**GAMUNU WIJETUNGE,** National Highway Traffic Safety Administration, U.S. Department of Transportation

Although the reviewers listed above provided many constructive comments and suggestions, they were not asked to endorse the content of the proceedings nor did they see the final draft before its release. The review of this proceedings was overseen by **ELI Y. ADASHI,** Brown University.

He was responsible for making certain that an independent examination of this proceedings was carried out in accordance with standards of the National Academies and that all review comments were carefully considered. Responsibility for the final content rests entirely with the rapporteurs and the National Academies.

# Contents

# Acronyms and Abbreviations

| | |
|---|---|
| ASPR | Assistant Secretary for Preparedness and Response |
| BARDA | Biomedical Advanced Research and Development Authority |
| CBRN | chemical, biological, radiological, or nuclear |
| CDC | U.S. Centers for Disease Control and Prevention |
| CIP | Critical Infrastructure Protection |
| DHS | U.S. Department of Homeland Security |
| DoD | U.S. Department of Defense |
| EHR | electronic health record |
| EMS | emergency medical services |
| FDA | U.S. Food and Drug Administration |
| FEMA | Federal Emergency Management Agency |
| FY | fiscal year |
| GHSA | Global Health Security Agenda |
| HHS | U.S. Department of Health and Human Services |
| HIE | health information exchange |
| HPP | Hospital Preparedness Program |

| | |
|---|---|
| ICS | incident command system |
| IHR | International Health Regulations |
| IRB | institutional review board |
| IT | information technology |
| | |
| JHSPH | Johns Hopkins Bloomberg School of Public Health |
| | |
| MCM | medical countermeasure |
| MERS-CoV | Middle Eastern respiratory syndrome coronavirus |
| MRC | Medical Reserve Corps |
| | |
| NACCHO | National Association of County & City Health Officials |
| NIH | National Institutes of Health |
| NLM | National Library of Medicine |
| | |
| PHEF | public health emergency fund |
| PHEMCE | Public Health Emergency Medical Countermeasure Enterprise |
| PHEP | Public Health Emergency Preparedness |
| PULSE | patient unified lookup system for emergencies |
| | |
| ROI | return on investment |
| | |
| USAID | U.S. Agency for International Development |
| | |
| WHO | World Health Organization |

# 1

# Introduction[1]

As the United States continues to adapt to a more digital, mobile, and interconnected world, health care and public health professionals have sought to better prepare for and respond to long-standing and emerging threats to the nation's health security. Health security is the collective effort to prevent, protect against, mitigate, respond to, and recover from the health consequences of natural, man-made, and technological disasters. Although substantial progress has been made in the past 15 years toward improving health care and public health systems and capacities for health security threats, many complex challenges persist, and often the nation's preparedness efforts are not sufficient. Given the transition to a new administration and Congress, the National Academies of Sciences, Engineering, and Medicine's Forum on Medical and Public Health Preparedness for Disasters and Emergencies (the forum) identified the present time as a unique opportunity to acknowledge these persistent issues; evaluate past, and perhaps inadequate, approaches to addressing them; and discuss intentional and innovative new solutions.

---

[1] The planning committee's role was limited to planning the workshop, and this Proceedings of a Workshop was prepared by the rapporteurs as a factual account of what occurred at the workshop. Statements, recommendations, and opinions expressed are those of individual presenters and participants and are not endorsed or verified by the National Academies of Sciences, Engineering, and Medicine and should not be construed as reflecting any group consensus.

**BOX 1-1**
**Workshop Objectives**

1. Examine challenges to medical and public health preparedness, response, and recovery in the context of topics such as global health security, communication and coordination, individual and community health resilience, and critical infrastructure protection.
2. Explore the direction of possible future policy actions and innovative approaches necessary to resolving these challenges.
3. Discuss possible opportunities for the Forum on Medical and Public Health Preparedness for Disasters and Emergencies and other stakeholders to contribute toward examining and addressing these challenges.

## ORGANIZATION OF THE WORKSHOP

To explore these persistent issues of preparedness, on March 8–9, 2017, the forum hosted a 2-day public workshop in Washington, DC, called Opportunities for the Future of Health Care and Public Health Preparedness, Response, and Recovery. Appendix A shows the workshop agenda and the workshop statement of task can be found in its entirety in Appendix B. Appendix C provides biographical sketches of the workshop speakers and moderators. The workshop objectives are highlighted in Box 1-1.

## ORGANIZATION OF THE PROCEEDINGS

These proceedings summarize the discussions and panel presentations that took place during the workshop. Chapter 2 provides an overview of the threat landscape as well as an overview of the complex network of stakeholders involved with U.S. health security. In Chapter 3, the threats and challenges that affect health care and public health critical infrastructure, data collection and use, program funding, and international disaster response cooperation are introduced. Chapter 4 continues to explore the challenges and underlying issues that have affected decision making and progress to date. Chapter 5 provides strategies for how health security initiatives might move forward. Finally, Chapter 6 highlights the importance of leveraging this transitional period.

# 2

# A Brief Overview of Health Security Threats and Programs

Tom Inglesby, director, Center for Health Security, Johns Hopkins Bloomberg School of Public Health (JHSPH), opened the workshop by noting that threats to U.S. health, safety, and security include not only major global and regional epidemics of emerging infectious diseases such as Ebola and Zika, but changes to the ways that known diseases, including dengue, chikungunya, yellow fever, and Middle Eastern respiratory syndrome coronavirus (MERS-CoV), are spreading throughout the world. Novel pandemic influenzas such as avian influenzas H5N1 and H7N9 are on the rise. The threat of chemical, biological, radiological, or nuclear (CBRN) attack is ever present, with sarin and chlorine gas used in terrorist attacks against civilians on a large scale. Inglesby remarked that natural, manmade, and technological disasters pose a serious threat to the nation's aging, and sometimes archaic, health care and public health infrastructures, as does the increasing frequency and severity of extreme weather events. These threats are compounded by probable changes to the health care system and a public health system that is chronically under financial stress across the federal, state, and local levels. Uncertainty prevails in key government entities involved in health security, despite the immediacy of the need to prepare for all types of threats.

Citing a Federal Emergency Management Agency (FEMA) report of crisis response and disaster resilience, Mitch Stripling, assistant commissioner, Bureau of Agency Preparedness and Response, New York City Health, emphasized that health security is a global problem of "increasing

**BOX 2-1**
**What Do Disasters Reveal?**

"The earliest disaster researchers actually talked a lot about how disasters are not actually extraordinary events. What disasters do and why disaster social scientists have so long been interested in these events is because of what they reveal. Some of the earliest writers working in this space in the 1950s said that what disasters serve to do is to strip away the veil that usually obscures the inner workings of society. By stripping away that veil, what it allows us to see is the underpinnings of society and it reveals to us what we value and sometimes what we do not value and also who we value and sometimes who we do not value."

—Lori Peek, author, *Children of Katrina*; Director, Natural Hazards Center and Professor of Sociology, University of Colorado

complexity and decreasing predictability in its operating environment."[1] There are more incidents, new and unfamiliar threats, more information, less time, new players and participants, and exceedingly high public expectations (see Box 2-1). Irwin Redlener, clinical professor, Health Policy and Management and Pediatrics, Columbia University, described how the scale and scope of preparedness not only for disasters, but for mega-disasters, have been inadequate for decades. Mega-disasters are so catastrophically eventful that they overwhelm local and regional capacities to really respond and mitigate their effects. He provided a set of defining criteria for mega-disasters, in descending order of priority: inability to manage immediate rescue of endangered survivors, significant backlog of victims unable to get appropriate medical care or other essential support, inability to protect vital infrastructure or prevent significant property destruction, and any level of societal breakdown or disorder.

To illustrate, Redlener described the consequences of two hypothetical mega-disaster scenarios. If a H5N1-type pandemic avian flu with a 30 percent attack rate occurred in New York City (population 8.2 million), there would likely be a hospitalization rate of 10 percent and a mortality rate among the infected of 2.5 percent. The potential realities of a 6-month flu season for a pandemic of this type would be 2.4 million people sick with

[1] *Crisis response and disaster resilience 2030: Forging strategic action in an age of uncertainty: Progress report highlighting the 2010–2011 insights of the strategic foresight initiative.* For more information, see https://www.fema.gov/media-library-data/20130726-1816-25045-5167/sfi_report_13.jan.2012_final.docx.pdf (accessed August 8, 2017).

avian flu (including 600,000 children) and 60,000 deaths (including 15,000 children) at a rate of more than 300 deaths each day. Hospitals would be overwhelmed by more than 200,000 admissions, and there would be a critical shortage of medical supplies such as vaccines, antiviral medications, hospital beds, ventilators, and other vital supplies. More importantly, he suggested, the cascading consequences would include problems such as schools closing, ill parents, potential quarantines, economic trouble, and little assistance from "the outside." In the scenario of a 10-kiloton improvised nuclear device detonation in Midtown Manhattan, according to Redlener, there would be 75,000–100,000 immediate fatalities and 300,000–500,000 surviving casualties requiring medical care, but there are less than 60,000 total staffed hospital beds in the entirety of New York state. He explained there are six main potential target cities for this type of attack—Los Angeles and San Francisco, California; Houston, Texas; Chicago, Illinois; New York City, New York; and Washington, District of Columbia—none of which are remotely prepared to deal with an improvised nuclear device. Redlener noted that "the capacity-to-need gap is enormous and insoluble as far we know right now."

Much work had been done in the areas of health security over the preceding 15 years, remarked Inglesby. The efforts have enabled many communities around the country to become more capable of caring for victims of more "normal" or anticipated disasters within some bounds. Inglesby noted that any health care system would be hard pressed to care for anything beyond a handful of highly contagious patients during a lethal epidemic or to care for large numbers of patients following major disasters. The goal should be to build health care and public health systems' capacity to care for and manage tens of thousands (or more) injured or infected people needing medical care during epidemics and catastrophes, remarked Inglesby.

Inglesby commented that to some extent, within the United States a national public health system that facilitates early detection of biological threats, controls epidemics, and responds to disasters has been built over many years. The United States and the world relies on the U.S. Centers for Disease Control and Prevention (CDC) during new epidemics (e.g., severe acute respiratory syndrome, H1N1, Ebola, and Zika). The United States relies on state and local public health officials for top-level scientific analysis and expertise on infectious diseases, surveillance programs and warning of new outbreaks, laboratory testing and safety, communicating risks to the public, medicine stockpiles, and community response programs, among others. At the state level, Inglesby remarked, capacity for preparedness and response is variable. In 2016, the National Health Security Preparedness

Index[2] revealed a national preparedness level ranking of 6.8 out of 10. This recent score demonstrates that although there is capacity in the system, there is plenty of room for improvement. Despite its crucial role, public health is chronically underfunded and lacks the resources for people and technology necessary to succeed, Inglesby remarked. In contrast, foundations are supporting public health like never before, and high numbers of young people are pursuing careers in public health (Leider et al., 2015; Prina, 2017).

According to Inglesby, the United States has the most impressive national ability to make new medical therapies, vaccines, and rapid diagnostics, including research and development for medical countermeasures (MCMs) for biological threats, antimicrobial resistance, pandemic flu, emerging diseases, and CBRN challenges. He attributed this ability to the efforts of the National Institutes of Health (NIH), the Office of the Assistant Secretary for Preparedness and Response (ASPR), the Biomedical Advanced Research and Development Authority (BARDA), the U.S. Food and Drug Administration (FDA), CDC, the U.S. Department of Defense (DoD), and the U.S. Department of Homeland Security (DHS) on the risk side, as well as universities and biopharmaceutical companies on the research and development side. He noted that the United States and much of the world has relied on this system to make MCMs during various past crises, including outbreaks such as 2001 anthrax, H5N1 bird flu, 2009 H1N1, the Ebola virus outbreak from 2013 to 2015, the ongoing Zika virus outbreak that started in 2015, and others. He described the Coalition for Epidemic Preparedness Innovations, an alliance to finance and coordinate the development of new vaccines to prevent and contain infectious disease epidemics, as a welcome development but noted that the development process still takes too long to make a difference during the most important period of a new outbreak. Flu is the best-case scenario, but in the past it has taken as long as 6 months after the discovery of a new flu pandemic for this system to produce an effective vaccine. For entirely novel threats, it can take a decade or longer, if at all, to develop new medicines and vaccines, unless the development process is already far along due to other reasons. Inglesby suggested aiming to achieve the goal set forth in the November 2016 President's Council of Advisors on Science and Technology report,[3] which called for the U.S. government to develop the national capacity (over the next 10 to 20 years) to make a new vaccine or medicine for any new biological threat within 6 months.

[2] See http://nhspi.org (accessed June 27, 2017).

[3] President's Council of Advisors on Science and Technology report, https://obamawhitehouse.archives.gov/sites/default/files/microsites/ostp/PCAST/pcast_biodefense_letter_report_final.pdf (accessed August 8, 2017).

A plethora of powerful new biotechnologies and transformative tools is on the horizon, according to Inglesby, with the potential to enormously benefit medicine, science, industry, and agriculture. Clustered, regularly interspaced, short palindromic repeats and their associated systems for editing, regulating, and targeting genomes is only one of the most visible tools emerging, and countries around the world are making billion-dollar investments. While we scan the horizon for new technologies and approaches to help prepare for new threats, he cautioned about the need to react wisely to potential adverse consequences biotechnologies will bring, such as novel, highly lethal, highly transmissible viruses that do not exist in nature. He suggested establishing international biosafety norms for laboratory work that has the potential to cause epidemics or great harm following accidental or deliberate laboratory release.

Maintaining norms against chemical, biological, and nuclear weapons through treaties and other means is more critical than ever, emphasized Inglesby, hence the importance of strengthening international health security to protect the United States and other countries and preventing the proliferation and use of chemical, biological, and nuclear weapons. Continued work on the international front to help contain outbreaks of infectious diseases outside of the United States is also critical, not only for reasons of ethics and expertise, but to prevent the spread of epidemics to the United States. As noted by Umair Shah, executive director of Harris County Public Health, global health security is essential to U.S. national security. The International Health Regulations (IHR) developed by the World Health Organization (WHO) in 2005 have established the norm that countries must be prepared to manage outbreaks of international importance, but only a small subset of countries is prepared to achieve this independently despite their commitment to IHR. The Global Health Security Agenda (GHSA) enlists talent and resources in many participating countries to help build a national-level epidemic response. The United States should continue to support and build on the progress of the GHSA, urged Inglesby.

Inglesby commented that many entities from both the public and private sectors have driving and supporting roles in U.S. health security. These include ASPR's Hospital Preparedness Program (HPP), BARDA, and the Healthcare and Public Health Sector Critical Infrastructure Protection (CIP) Program; DHS's Office of Health Affairs National Biosurveillance Integration Center and BioWatch; the National Disaster Medical System; CDC's Public Health Emergency Preparedness (PHEP) Program; FDA; NIH; DoD; the Medical Reserve Corps (MRC); nongovernmental organizations, such as Healthcare Ready, the National Association of County & City Health Officials (NACCHO), the Association of State and Territorial Health Officials, the Council on State and Territorial Epidemiologists, the Association of Public Health Laboratories, the National Association of Chain Drug

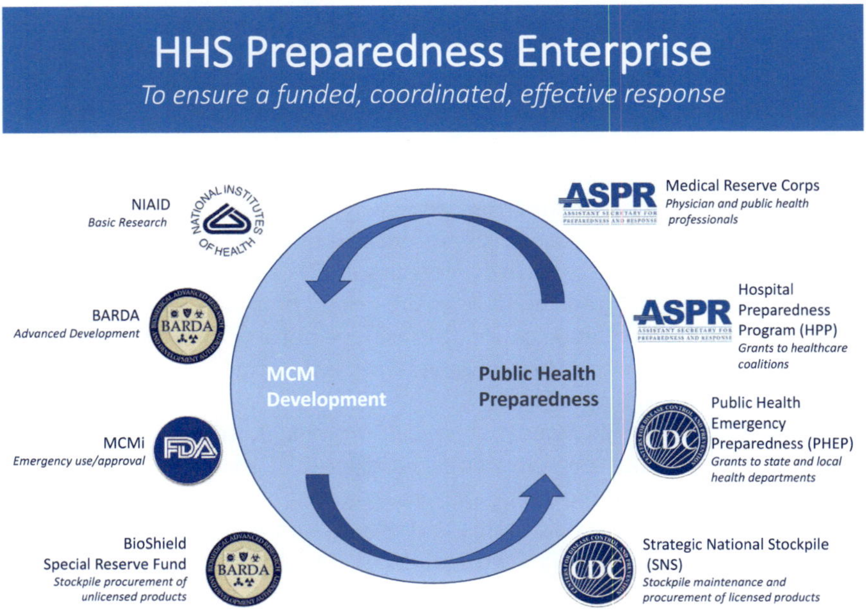


**FIGURE 2-1** HHS Preparedness Enterprise.
NOTE: ASPR = Assistant Secretary for Preparedness and Response; BARDA = Biomedical Advanced Research and Development Authority; CDC = U.S. Centers for Disease Control and Prevention; FDA = U.S. Food and Drug Administration; HHS = U.S. Department of Health and Human Services; MCMi = Medical Countermeasures Initiative; NIAID = National Institute of Allergy and Infectious Diseases.
SOURCES: Hanen presentation, March 9, 2017; East End Group (eastendgrp.com).

Stores, and the American Red Cross; and local and state health departments, health care coalitions, and private health care system programs serving communities throughout the nation.

Laura Hanen, chief, Government Affairs, NACCHO, provided an overview of the U.S. Department of Health and Human Services (HHS) Preparedness Enterprise, which aims to ensure a funded, coordinated, effective response to health threats across many of these entities (see Figure 2-1).

Maria Julia Marinissen, director, Division of International Health Security, Office of Policy and Planning, ASPR, HHS, described how the 2006 Pandemic and All-Hazards Preparedness Act and 2013 Reauthorization Act created and established ASPR leadership in national and international preparedness and response initiatives and activities. Other duties required by ASPR include providing personnel, countermeasures, coordination, and logistics surrounding disaster response. HHS leads federal public health

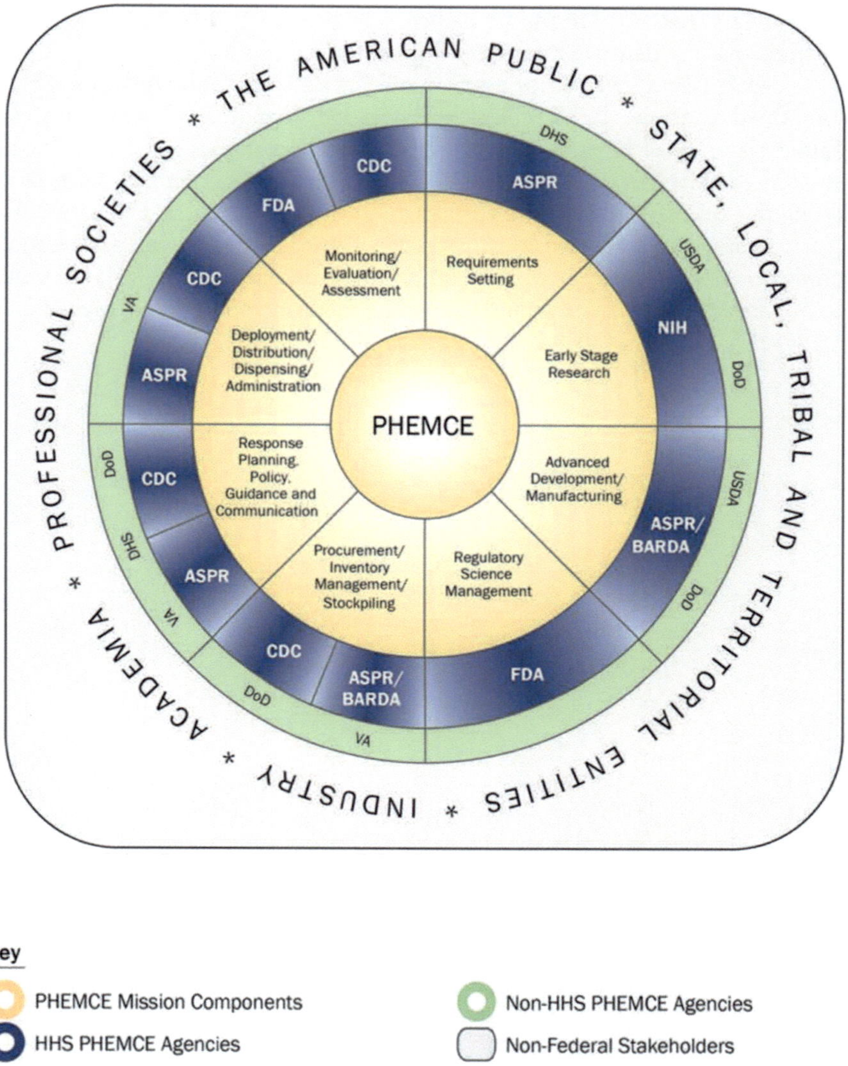


**FIGURE 2-2** PHEMCE.
NOTE: ASPR = Assistant Secretary for Preparedness and Response; BARDA = Biomedical Advanced Research and Development Authority; CDC = U.S. Centers for Disease Control and Prevention; DHS = U.S. Department of Homeland Security; DoD = U.S. Department of Defense; FDA = U.S. Food and Drug Administration; HHS = U.S. Department of Health and Human Services; NIH = National Institutes of Health; PHEMCE = Public Health Emergency Medical Countermeasures Enterprise; USDA = U.S. Department of Agriculture; VA = U.S. Department of Veterans Affairs.
SOURCES: Hu-Primmer presentation, March 8, 2017; ASPR, 2017.

and medical response to public health emergencies and National Response Framework incidents (Emergency Support Function #8).

Jean Hu-Primmer, senior advisor, CBRN and Pandemic Influenza, FDA, explained that the Public Health Emergency Medical Countermeasures Enterprise (PHEMCE) is also led by ASPR and comprises HHS entities such as FDA, NIH, BARDA, and CDC. PHEMCE coordinates with DoD, DHS, the U.S. Department of Veterans Affairs (VA), the U.S. Department of Agriculture, and state and local public health officials, as well as hospitals, clinical networks, and medical product manufacturers in the private sector to advance the nation's capacity for public health response (see Figure 2-2).

# 3

# Proposed Priorities and Persistent Challenges Related to Health Security

There are a range of threats to the nation's health security that have the potential to cause widespread disruption and damage to human health, the economy, and society at large. As noted by Inglesby, great strides have been made toward improving health care and public health systems and capacities across the public and private sectors. In this chapter, experts representing a variety of sectors discuss their perspectives on the priorities and persistent challenges related to health security, focusing specifically on health care and public health critical infrastructure protection, data collection and use, funding for health security programs, preparedness for global health emergencies, and vulnerable populations and community resilience. Ensuring a robust health care and public health sector will greatly advance the nation's ability to respond and recover when faced with a health security threat.

## HEALTH CARE AND PUBLIC HEALTH CRITICAL INFRASTRUCTURE PROTECTION

Laura Wolf, chief, CIP Branch, ASPR, HHS, provided a definition of critical infrastructure as "systems and assets, whether physical or virtual, so vital to the United States that their incapacitation or destruction would have a debilitating impact on national security, economic security, public health or safety, or any combination of those matters."[1] She emphasized that critical infrastructure encompasses not only physical buildings, but the

[1] § 1016(e) of the USA Patriot Act of 2001 (42 U.S.C. § 5195c(e)).

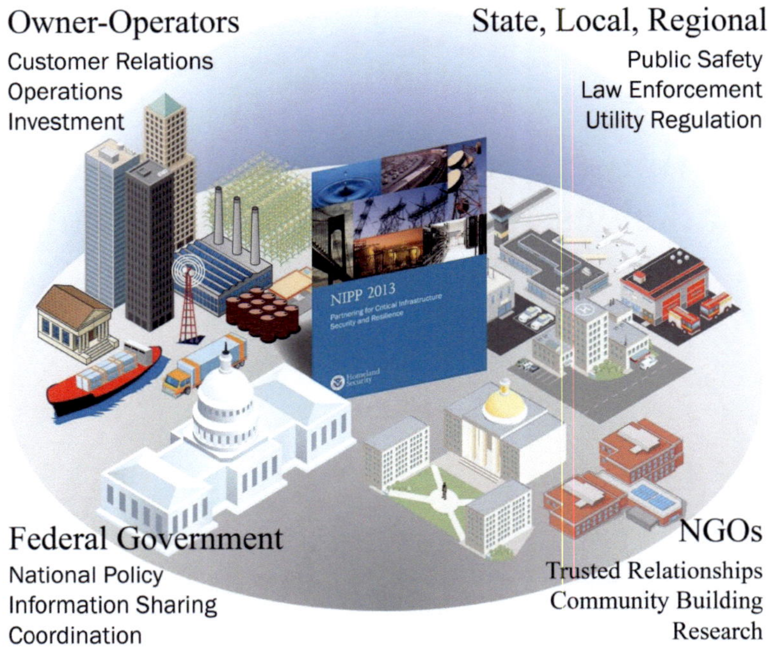


**FIGURE 3-1** Health care and public health CIP foundation.
NOTE: NGO = nongovernmental organization.
SOURCES: Wolf presentation, March 8, 2017; U.S. Department of Homeland Security.

systems and assets that are fundamentally required to perform the functions needed for public health and safety.[2] She reflected that 2.5 million people per day access health care and public health critical infrastructure.

Wolf described the national-level health care and public health CIP foundation as an instructive model of partnership to promote capacity building and preparedness (see Figure 3-1).

The HHS/ASPR CIP Program works with government and private-sector partners to enhance the security and resilience of the health care and public health sector by mitigating risks to critical infrastructure.[3]

---

[2] For example, Wolf noted, going to a medical office for treatment in a facility that has power and water; where staff take health insurance information and access electronic health records; where a doctor uses lab tests to make a diagnosis; and if treatment is needed, where prescriptions are easily transmitted to a pharmacy that has the needed supplies in stock.

[3] More information about the partnership and the 2015–2018 health care and public health sector–specific plan is available at www.phe.gov/cip (accessed August 8, 2017).

This voluntary partnership is not tied to regulation or funding and seeks to address crosscutting issues not only in the health care field, but also to examine its interdependencies (such as power, water, transportation, and research and development) and to determine ways to better respond to all types of activities. Joint working groups[4] of the Government Coordinating Council, which is composed of public-sector components with an interest and role in health care and public health sector critical infrastructure security and resilience, and the Sector Coordinating Council, which is a self-organized and self-governed council of health care and public health private-sector partners,[5] are convened routinely as part of the Critical Infrastructure Partnership Advisory Council and are exempt from the Federal Advisory Committee Act. Although activities are communicated to the public, business-sensitive information is protected, which builds trust among partners.[6] CIP's structure connects it with 15 other sectors of critical infrastructure and during a response, FEMA's National Business Emergency Operations Center brings these sectors together.

The essential components of critical infrastructure, according to Wolf, are "staff, stuff, systems, and space." *Staff* includes office personnel, doctors, truck drivers, manufacturers, information technology (IT) security, and researchers. *Stuff* covers, for example, rapid flu tests, gloves, swabs, drugs, blood supply, and vaccines. *Systems* comprise transportation, health insurance, health IT, supply chains, research and development, and funding. *Space* involves medical and public health buildings, security, power and water, pharmacies, distribution hubs, and laboratories. Wolf also described the multiple health care and public health subsectors at play in critical infrastructure: direct patient care, pharmacies, laboratories and blood banks, health IT, medical materials (distributors, manufacturers, and materials managers at facilities), plans and payers, mass fatality management, state and local public health departments and related associations, and federal response and program offices.

Oscar Alleyne, NACCHO, noted that from a local health department lens, the "staff" element of critical infrastructure means ensuring there are enough trained staff on the ground to respond during an emergency while maintaining continuity of operations with regular programs and services. Dave Dyjack, executive director, National Environmental Health Association, used the environmental health workforce as an example of the benefits gained by bringing the right people to the table in the preparedness,

[4] Joint working groups include a Risk Management Working Group and Cybersecurity Working Group.

[5] Sector Coordinating Council workgroups include Activate Shooter, Situational Cybersecurity, Legislation, and Supply Chain.

[6] The CIP Advisory Council charter is available at https://www.dhs.gov/sites/default/files/publications/cipac-charter-11-30-16-508.pdf (accessed August 8, 2017).

response, and recovery enterprise. He recounted that a FEMA call after Hurricane Matthew for workers and volunteers in October 2016 included a wide range of sectors but that environmental health professionals who work with these sectors daily were not included in the call. "The challenge that we have is that we don't invite environmental health professionals to the table early. We don't recognize them as a resource," he said.

Dyjack stressed that public health is environmental health and that the environmental health sector comprises the largest part of the public health workforce.[7] Environmental health professionals are in the field every day, understand the culture and the risks, and in many cases have locally funded data-collection systems in place. Environmental health also needs to be part of continuous quality improvement issues, he argued. As innovative techniques are introduced, the environmental health and clinical care sectors should work together systematically to validate, assess, and measure intervention effectiveness. He commended the University of Nebraska's National Ebola Training and Education Center for inviting environmental health and industrial hygienists to the table early on to address issues related to the transmission of Ebola in those environments.

Wolf illustrated the evolving threat to the supply chain of health care and public health critical infrastructure. Different products, supply chains, people, and networks were factors in the range of responses to evolving threats over the past 10 years. The 2009–2010 H1N1 pandemic highlighted the need for syringes, needles, and masks. The 2013 saline shortages called attention to gaps in access to saline products in the event of an emergency. The 2014 Ebola virus crisis in western Africa showcased the need for access to personal protective equipment in the midst of hoarding and supplying challenges. The 2016 Zika outbreak, which focused on prevention, called attention to gaps in vector control. Wolf emphasized that each of those responses to evolving threats was contingent on access to supplies through public–private partnerships. Partnering in the health care and public health enterprise requires coordination among and between the public sector (e.g., VA, DoD, CDC, the Association of State and Territorial Health Officials, NACCHO), private sector (e.g., Healthcare Industry Distributors Association, Consumer Specialty Products Association, and the Medical Device Manufacturers Association), and coordinating groups (e.g., PHEMCE, the Global Supply Network for Pandemic Preparedness and Response, and the All-Hazards Consortium).

Gregg Margolis, director, Division of Healthcare System Policy, HHS, provided an overview of the substantial and cascading impacts that disasters have on health care and public health systems. He explained that al-

[7] Dyjack cited the Bureau of Labor Statistics and said there are about 88,000 environmental scientists in the country. The next closest group is public health nurses at around 40,000 to 45,000.

though each disaster is different, they have certain common characteristics. A rapid influx of patients with unscheduled needs can stress health care systems in ways no other events can. Disasters cause many acute injuries in people who are displaced from their regular sources of care and seek care in emergency departments without access to their medical records. Large numbers of people affected by a disaster may be from vulnerable populations and/or have chronic comorbidities that exacerbate and lengthen care requirements. Evacuations and interruptions in the normal health care infrastructure due to disasters can also debilitate health care systems, he noted. As seen in the Ebola and Zika epidemics, disasters give rise to many challenges related to information needs, such as disseminating information and clinical algorithms that are evolving during an event to clinicians providing care and making decisions beyond their normal responsibilities.

John Hick, medical director, Emergency Preparedness, Hennepin County Medical Center, emphasized that the "space," or physical infrastructure, is a fundamental necessity—for example, power and water are required to provide care. He outlined a set of "mission-essential functions" for physical infrastructure and facilities: structure, utilities, heating and air-conditioning, air handling, medical gases, telecommunications (Internet, and IT systems), electronic health records (EHRs), medical supplies, transport, nutrition, pharmacies, laboratories, radiology, security, laundry, human resources, and environmental health. Hick warned that risk is endemic in the United States, with large populations living in areas that experience significant natural hazards and others living in areas that are part of large infrastructure networks (e.g., electricity) at risk of technological hazards. Hick expressed grave concerns about the reliability of the aging utilities infrastructure in the United States. For example, if a coronal mass ejection occurred matching the May 1921 geomagnetic storm level (not even at a greater magnitude like the Carrington event, a solar storm in 1859), then 130 million people would lose power for weeks or months at a time, mainly across the eastern half of the United States and the Pacific northwest (see Figure 3-2).

Hick explained that the level of event in this model would have a dramatic impact on health care and public health critical infrastructure. Electricity has no specific sites for public access because it is a public service, not a private enterprise (similar to health care, but more widely distributed). He explained that even short-term blackouts cause consistent cascading failures in infrastructure and systems.[8]

Hick also warned that trends for billion-dollar climate disasters are

---

[8] For example, Hick described a person on electricity-dependent oxygen at home who must come into the hospital and vendor chains falling apart because gasoline is not available. Hospitals are not used to running at 100 percent on their generators and they usually do not have appropriate generator support to back up their HVAC systems.

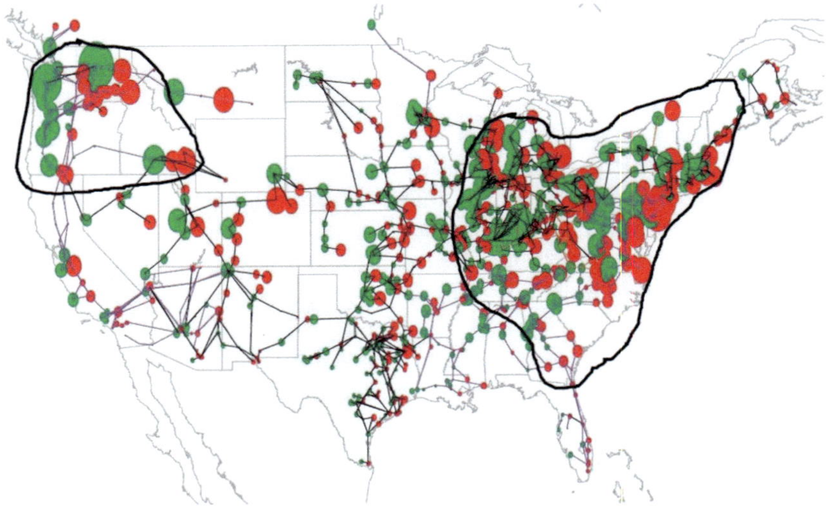

**FIGURE 3-2** Model of 1921-level geomagnetic storm scenario.
NOTE: The regions outlined are susceptible to system collapse due to geomagnetically induced current. The impacts would involve populations in excess of 130 million.
SOURCES: Hick presentation, March 8, 2017; Geomagnetic Storms and Their Impacts on the U.S. Power Grid, January 2010.

increasing, with four of the five most powerful hurricanes in recorded history occurring within the last decade. As ocean waters warm, storms will become more intense and will remain intense farther northward than ever before (see Figure 3-3).

Presenters and participants identified persistent difficulties related to assessing, protecting, and strengthening the existing health care and public health critical infrastructure, as well as strengthening stakeholder engagement in national-level discussions about health security. Rear Admiral Carmen T. Maher, acting assistant commissioner for Counterterrorism Policy, FDA, suggested that critical infrastructure sustainability requires ensuring accountability, objectively evaluating systems in place to adapt or augment obsolescence or ineffective pieces, and investing in integrating preparedness and response components in day-to-day and other systems across the public and private sectors. She noted that the systems carrying out day-to-day safety, efficacy, and data collection also have both the funding capability and structure to surge up and serve during emergencies.

Deborah Levy, professor and interim chair, Epidemiology Department, University of Nebraska Medical Center, College of Public Health, noted that preparedness and response are often considered too separate and distinct from the day-to-day operation of health care and public health critical infrastructure, especially in terms of funding, but she suggested that those basic, everyday needs must be met before thinking about and devoting resources for preparedness or emergency response. David Abramson, professor, Center for Global Health, New York University, agreed about the need for health and human services systems to respond to community needs, both routine and during an emergency.

Roy Alson, Wake Forest School of Medicine, pointed out that communities with health care systems that are able to provide effective care on a routine basis are better prepared to respond to disasters. However, he explained that many components of health care and public health critical infrastructure are situated in systems that are stressed and often inadequate on a daily basis. Asking leadership and the public to commit more resources to strengthen the system for potential disasters in the face of daily systemic insufficiencies presents a conflict, he warned, and surmounting it will require taking a broader view and working to fix the entire system: "As we talk about preparedness and our ability to respond to unplanned or even unanticipated events, we must do it in the entire context of how to manage our day-to-day disasters."

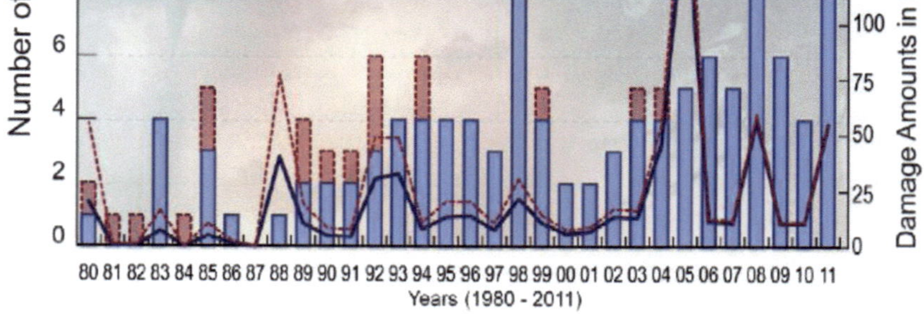


FIGURE 3-3 Cost-adjusted billion-dollar weather and climate disasters over time (1980–2011).
SOURCES: Hick presentation, March 8, 2017; U.S. Billion-dollar Weather and Climate Disasters: Data Sources, Trends, Accuracy and Biases. Introduction (p. 338). Natural Hazards, June 2013, Volume 67, Issue 2, p. 338.

John Osborn, operations administrator, Department of Practice Administration, Mayo Clinic, commented on awareness and recognition of the importance of health care and public health among the other sectors of critical infrastructure. He noted that because the systems are so tightly integrated, attempting to separate out one problem to solve will not accomplish much. He also remarked on the extent to which other sectors of the economy do not realize they require health care services and further suggested that spending a fraction of the investments being made in those other sectors on public health could potentially relieve the overburdened public health system. Laura Runnels, LAR Consulting,[9] noted the persistent struggle of clearly demonstrating and communicating the value of health care and public health to the public, the private sector, and the government. Dyjack highlighted the near absence of recognition of public health. For example, no one contracted and died of Ebola virus in the United States during the worldwide pandemic, but this successful solution was not recognized or celebrated as it would be in other professions.

## DATA COLLECTION AND USE

Margolis explained that data collected from a disaster comes in different forms that include EHRs, but also draw from "operational data, administrative data, scheduling data, workforce data, inventory management data." Public health departments are effective when it comes to technical components of data interoperability platforms, noted Lee Stevens, director, Office of State Policy, Office of the National Coordinator for Health IT, HHS. He continued that problems arise with "consistent data formats and particularly around data quality."

Stripling gave the example of the New York City health department's use and value of data in their preparedness planning and, ultimately, evaluation. He commented that "in the city health department, what we are doing is we are laying out all of the consequences that we know we are fighting against. . . . It is creating a big data set of thousands of activities literally that we performed over the last decade. But by putting those in data, we make them queryable-like data, tagging them like data. We are talking [about an] all hazards data warehouse that we can then connect to all the other data that we are dealing with. When we run our preparedness cycle, we base it on those activities. And in response, we can evaluate those activities."

Hu-Primmer described efforts to address one aspect, a comprehensive, governmentwide coordinated capability to monitor and assess MCM use

[9] Laura Runnels is a consultant facilitator hired by the National Academies to assist with group process and to offer her own observations on themes as a participant of the workshop.

(including safety, compliance, and clinical benefit) through data collection and analysis during and after an emergency event. These data would enable better assessment and decision making during both present and future public health responses. Such an effort requires a comprehensive governmentwide centralized and coordinated capability—a "middle lane"—to bridge the gap between limited (or a lack of) data collection during a public emergency and traditional randomized controlled trial data collection. This middle lane is important, she explained, because it is nearly impossible to rely on traditional data collection; it is extraordinarily difficult to execute randomized controlled trials in the absence of an emergency, let alone during an emergency. Limited anecdotal data or emerging information are plagued by questions over the reliability and robustness of that data. The middle lane will be required to carry out coordinated, predefined, predetermined data collection and to create abbreviated case reports for prospectively defined fields and nested protocols. She reported that the U.S. government is already taking steps to establish this middle lane by using the "crawl-walk-run" paradigm: define the needed dataset; develop a simple protocol to collect the needed dataset; send the protocol to local institutional review boards (IRBs) for review; develop reliance agreements between local IRBs and a centralized IRB; and then preposition the IRB-approved protocol and exercise on a yearly basis.

Margolis noted that in today's environment, health care executives have better situational awareness about what is going on within their facilities than ever before. However, this information is not routinely shared due to several reasons (i.e., the information is proprietary). As a result, Margolis remarked, "We have an amazing blind spot in our health care system: virtually no health care situational awareness. There is no one that has a view of what is going on in the overall health care system. We do not really understand what the capacity, capability, and stress on health care systems are every day or during disasters. . . . If you can't do it every day, you won't be able to do it during a disaster." He defined health care situational awareness as understanding the capabilities, capacity, and stress on health care organizations in a given geographical area.[10]

Multiple participants highlighted the challenge of striking the right balance between having enough versus too much data. Runnels observed that public health does not always have the type of data it needs; for example, most local health departments do not have access to EHRs. Furthermore,

[10] Margolis explained that this gap in situational awareness is evident during an emergency, when state, local, and emergency management need real-time, detailed information about hospitals: "What hospitals are open/closed? Who is evacuating/sheltering-in-place? What hospitals are on auxiliary power? At capacity, near capacity, how many more patients can they take? What is the critical care capacity? Pediatrics? How many ventilators do they have? Do they have adequate supplies? What is running out? Are the staff able to get to work?"

she suggested that lack of data may lead other entities to perceive public health as vulnerable, and this perception may undercut public health's authority and involvement in a community. She also commented on the challenges of data timeliness and accuracy: "Either we do not have enough, or it is not coming to us quickly enough, or we have too much and it is changing all the time." Stripling characterized this national-level problem as the "data rabbit hole": there are exponentially increasing amounts of data available, but too much data are useless and largely go unanalyzed. Data can also become overwhelming and obfuscate elements of a community's response, he warned.

Redlener cautioned against overemphasizing data needs for problems that may not need more data to solve, because it can become a tempting screen to hide behind and avoid facing other big challenges. For example, in the hypothetical case of a 10-kiloton improvised nuclear device hitting New York City requiring the accommodation of 50,000 evacuees, he argued that data do not contribute to a macro-level understanding of what evacuees need or how to carry out the evacuation in practice. He argued that many issues related to preparedness, response, and recovery are not amenable to more information or research, but conceded that data are important operationally.[11]

The democratization of data, Stripling suggested, can also impede a response: "We no longer live in a world where we can follow data to a solution. It is not functional. . . . We must first understand our mission and then hit the data within it." He cautioned that "dropping the data in the middle of the response" can have serious ramifications, because the democratization of data can lead to misinterpretation by nonexperts. For example, if epidemiologists use data to create a map with a circle on it during a response, it may be perceived by the public, policy makers, and media as a threat rather than a tool for localizing the source of injury: "Everybody thinks that is where people are going to get hurt. That makes it a political objective, not an investigation object." In some cases, according to Stripling, it is necessary to confine data to the epidemiologists' sphere because only their expert judgment is useful.

Karl Schmitt, bParati, noted that the challenge of "chasing the data point" can overwhelm and waste limited resources. Redlener pointed to this as another example of the "data rabbit hole"—having large amounts of data without a structured mission to operationalize that data. He illustrated this challenge with a hypothetical situation: during a large disaster, responders have data about a person who is oxygen dependent, but no

---

[11] For example, Redlener noted data can be useful in determining what a hospital is doing or not doing, what it can accommodate, or where its capacities are being stressed in the midst of an acute emergency in a particular location.

knowledge of the clinical outcomes. If the person does not answer the phone, "Is she lying dead on the floor? Is she perfectly safe and evacuated? We do not know. We go to knock on her door. Her power is out. There is no answer. Do we break down the door? If we find her, do we bring her food? Do we prioritize that person because we have data over another place that we do not have any data about? These are the choices that data lead us to." Without a clearly established mission, data can effectively paralyze the response. He explained that having a data point about a person does not show one survivor, it shows all the potential survivors who could express that data point: "An oxygen-dependent woman, who might be fine, might not be fine, might have family, might not have family, might have support, or might not have support."

Several participants also emphasized weaknesses in the system's current ability to collect, validate, and disseminate data on risk and threat information during emergencies, to integrate advances in research and technology, and to use and collect electronic health data before, during, and after an emergency response. Stacy Arnesen, National Library of Medicine (NLM), NIH, suggested a set of key questions to consider about the role of data in this space: "What is the purpose of data? How do we ensure data match/help meet the mission? What data are needed? What to collect? What to save/preserve? What tools will assist with interoperability, integration, and analysis?" Maher explained that just as key decisions are different in different emergencies, so are the kinds of data needed to inform those decisions and that the challenge is to find the quickest way to collect and analyze data, look at outputs, and communicate findings. Dylan George, associate director, B.Next, In-Q-Tel, and former senior advisor, Biological Threats Defense, Office of Science and Technology Policy, White House, suggested the need to improve quantitative analytics and data sharing for improved decision making.[12] He also noted that data sharing within the federal government, at the state and local levels, and within academia lacks breadth, effectiveness, and nimbleness. Wolf remarked that health care and response are data driven, but data protection and privacy concerns can impede information sharing.

Ongoing broad challenges, according to Levy, include developing better health systems informatics, establishing a common operating picture, and addressing information-sharing needs. Michael G. Kurilla, director, Office of BioDefense, Research Resources, and Translational Research, and associate director for BioDefense Product Development, Division of Microbiology and Infectious Diseases, National Institute of Allergy and Infectious Diseases, NIH, HHS, suggested the need to better integrate and leverage evolv-

---

[12] George noted that during H1N1 modeling was not very useful (and in fact confused the response), but during Ebola it had a positive impact and was used to inform decision making.

ing technology. Maher noted the challenge of building technical and human resource infrastructures that can manage all the different data streams and help to prioritize and select the most relevant ones. Redlener highlighted the hour-to-hour dynamic reality of the collection and accuracy of data (e.g., last week's functional disability list is no longer current), which makes it difficult to operationalize data and carry out operational planning. He suggested that a key challenge in addressing this issue will be determining how often data need to be collected from a functional perspective.

Rajiv Ramnath, director, National Science Foundation, raised the issue of the research agenda, research gaps, and whether the need is to collect new types of information or to integrate the information that is already available. Jesse L. Goodman, professor of medicine, Georgetown University, also remarked on the challenge of defining and disseminating science gaps and the research agenda. Levy noted that rigorous, evidence-based evaluation and study design tend to be ad hoc in preparedness as compared to other parts in the public health arena.

## FUNDING FOR HEALTH SECURITY PROGRAMS

Several workshop participants discussed and explored the challenges in financing and sustainability of health security and preparedness. Dara Alpert Lieberman, senior government relations manager, Trust for America's Health, reported that her organization's latest annual preparedness report, *Ready or Not? Protecting the Public's Health from Diseases, Disasters, and Bioterrorism*,[13] discusses an established pattern within public health financing. Overall baseline public health funding is cut, and then a new crisis arises for which Congress may provide supplemental funding; once the crisis passes from national attention, the system reverts to budget cuts. Hick advised, "You get what you pay for in the end with public health and with emergency preparedness. If you don't want to invest, that is fine, but with no investment there is no return. There will be failures."

Disease can spread nearly anywhere within 24 hours through the global aviation network, and both natural disasters and terrorist events can hit with no warning, cautioned Lieberman. She explained that the common factor in all types of crisis events is that time is critical for mounting a robust, immediate public health response. Such a response requires having access to funding, supplies, and people in place as soon as possible after event onset. However, she explained that for various political reasons, Congress generally does not move quickly enough in funding an immediate response. For example, it only took 1 day for Congress to respond to then President

[13] See http://www.healthyamericans.org/assets/files/TFAH2012ReadyorNot10.pdf (accessed August 8, 2017).

George W. Bush's request for a Hurricane Katrina supplement, but nearly 8 months lapsed between then President Barack Obama's initial request for Zika response money and the final Congressional approval (see Figure 3-4).

Lieberman explained that public health funding for preparedness is tied into larger overall federal budget and debt reduction conversations. Fiscal year (FY) 2018 is a sequester year with tight funding caps, so the macro-level funding issues will have a cascade effect on all nondiscretionary programs. Hanen reported that nondefense discretionary spending in FY 2018 will reach a record low as a mere one percent of the gross domestic product, with data going back to 1962. Despite this, she noted, President Donald Trump will potentially propose a $54 billion increase for defense programs, with a commensurate decrease in nondefense discretionary programs (see Figure 3-5).

Hanen suggested there may be a silver lining, in that there are policy makers who recognize the need for providing funds for public health programs and are searching for solutions to fund the Preparedness Enterprise. For example, she quoted Chairman Kohl of the Labor–HHS Appropriations Subcommittee in the House of Representatives as opposing President Trump's approach of a commensurate cut in nondefense spending with a commensurate increase in defense spending, and stating that CDC is as

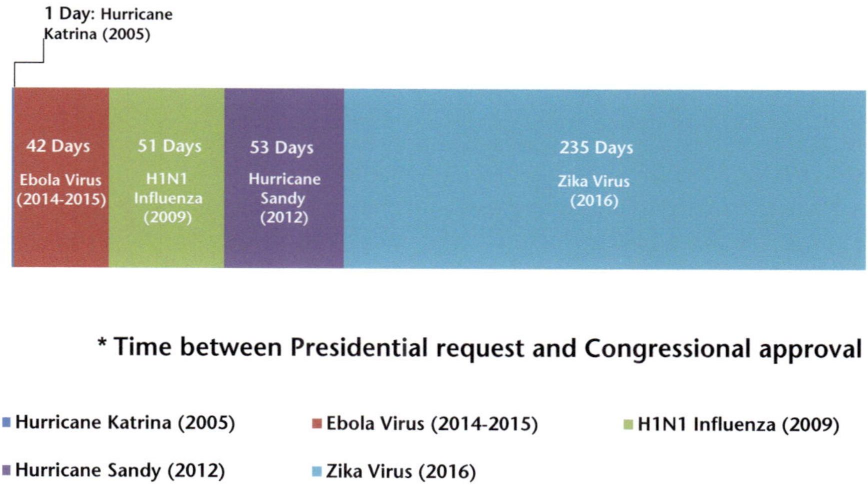


FIGURE 3-4 Delays in funding for public health emergencies.
SOURCES: Lieberman presentation, March 9, 2017; reprinted from *Ready or Not?: Protecting the Public from Diseases, Disasters, and Bioterrorism*, http://healthyamericans.org/reports/readyornot2016 (accessed October 3, 2017).

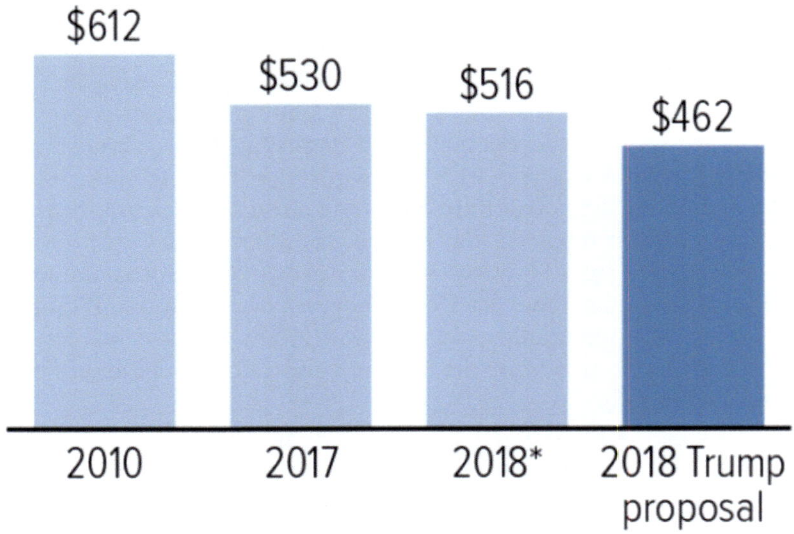


FIGURE 3-5 FY 2018 presidential budget: non-defense appropriations would fall under Trump plan.
NOTES: Measured in billions of 2018 dollars; * = funding level set in 2011 Budget Control Act, which establishes sequestration cuts; data source = CBPP analysis of data from the Congressional Budget Office and the Office of Management and Budget.
SOURCES: Hanen presentation, March 9, 2017; reprinted from the Center on Budget and Policy Priorities (cbpp.org).

important to defending the average American as the DoD: "You are a lot more likely to die in a pandemic than a terrorist attack."[14]

Hanen provided an overview of funding trends in the enterprise through FY 2016. She explained that most health departments receive money through their state health departments, with 55 percent of local health departments relying solely on federal funding. There has been a 34 percent reduction in PHEP funding over the last decade, and she noted that this lack of sustained and robust funding presents problems when issues arise and Congress must be asked for resources (see Figure 3-6).

Cuts to the ASPR's HPP in recent years have also hampered the pursuit of robust health system preparedness with health care coalitions, noted Hanen. Funding was decreased by $104 million (29 percent) in FY 2014

[14] When asked about the 12 percent cut to CDC's budget as a result of the Prevention to Public Health Fund, Chairman Kohl said, "Having a robustly funded CDC is very much in the national interest." He also put in a $300 million bill in 2017 for an infectious disease rapid response fund in CDC.

and by 54 percent over the last decade, depending on the benchmark in the federal budget bill (see Figure 3-7).

Two-thirds of the MRC units, another piece of the Preparedness Enterprise, are based in local health departments. Hanen explained that MRC units include volunteers who work with local departments to extend capacity by staffing points of dispensation, such as flu clinics. MRC funding has also been cut over time, including a $3 million cut in FY 2016 from FY 2015, representing a 40 percent decrease from FY 2006 (see Figure 3-8).

The Strategic National Stockpile will need continued resources to maintain, replenish, and provide additional licensed products to the stockpile, according to Hanen. These are discretionarily appropriated programs that require "going back to the well" annually (see Figure 3-9).

BARDA, which is housed within ASPR, facilitates the development and purchase of therapies, vaccines, and diagnostic tools for public health medical emergencies. Hanen noted that BARDA was originally funded through an advanced appropriation of a transfer from Project BioShield that expired

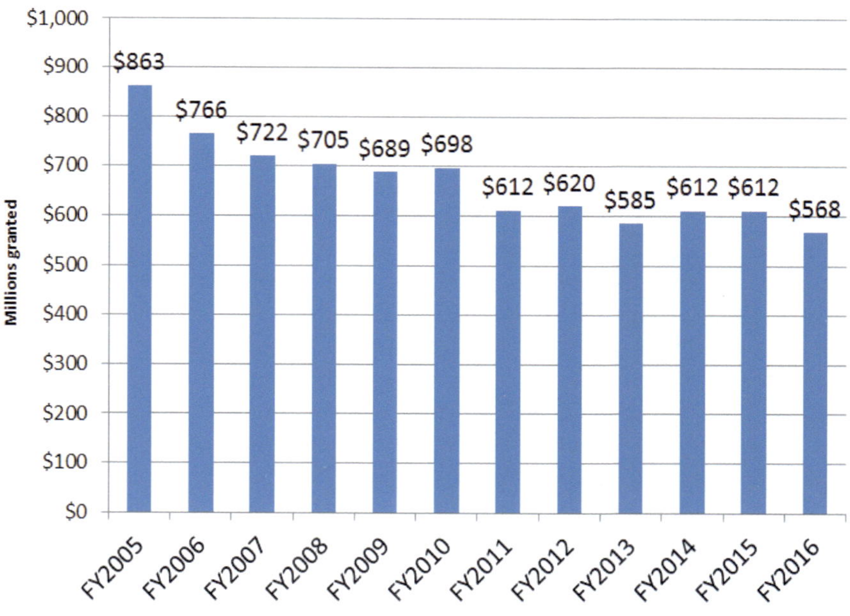


**FIGURE 3-6** CDC PHEP funding to health departments (FY 2005–FY 2016).
NOTES: Measured by $ in millions granted; 34 percent cut in funding since FY 2005.
SOURCES: Hanen presentation, March 9, 2017; NACCHO based on funding awards.

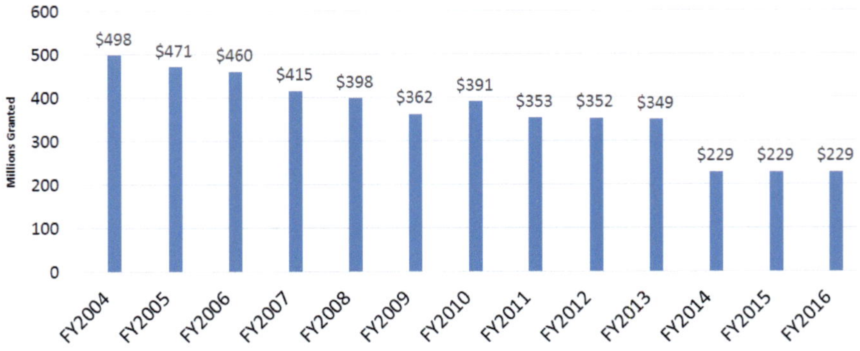


**FIGURE 3-7** ASPR HPP funding to health departments (FY 2004–FY 2016).
NOTES: Measured by $ in millions granted; 54 percent reduction since FY 2004.
SOURCES: Hanen presentation, March 9, 2017; NACCHO based on funding awards.

at the end of FY 2013. Currently, BARDA is also reliant on the annual budget appropriations process. She emphasized that during tight budget times with budget caps, the appropriations process amounts to a zero-sum game that pits all these programs against one another for funding.

Inglesby and others endorsed the concept of using the public health emergency fund (PHEF) as a means to quickly fund an emergency response. Lieberman provided an overview of the potential benefits and drawbacks of this solution. She noted that some have likened PHEF to FEMA for public health emergencies, but her organization, Trust for America's Health, views it as a surge fund to supplement rather than supplant. This distinction means it complements but does not replace sufficient, stable funding and is meant to serve as a bridge between the onset of an emergency and (if necessary) supplemental funding. She explained that under existing authority (1983), the Secretary of HHS would control the no-year fund and be required to report to Congress on how the money is spent. However, no money has been provided to the existing PHEF since FY 1999. She suggested that the lack of designated funding may be one of the reasons why more public health emergencies are not declared. However, she noted that there have been proposals in Congress during spring 2017 that could address this problem. She highlighted the bipartisan Public Health Emergency Response and Accountability Act (Senators Bill Cassidy and Brian Schatz), which includes a funding formula that looks at the past 14 years of public health emergency spending (approximately $1.5 billion to start). Funding would be controlled at the HHS department level and could be used

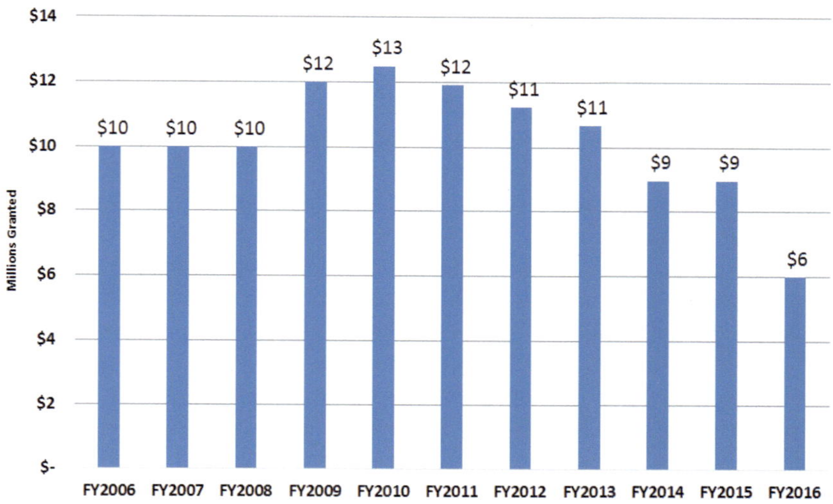


**FIGURE 3-8** MRC funding (FY 2006–FY 2016).
NOTES: Measured by $ in millions; 40 percent reduction since FY 2006.
SOURCES: Hanen presentation, March 9, 2017; NACCHO based on funding awards.

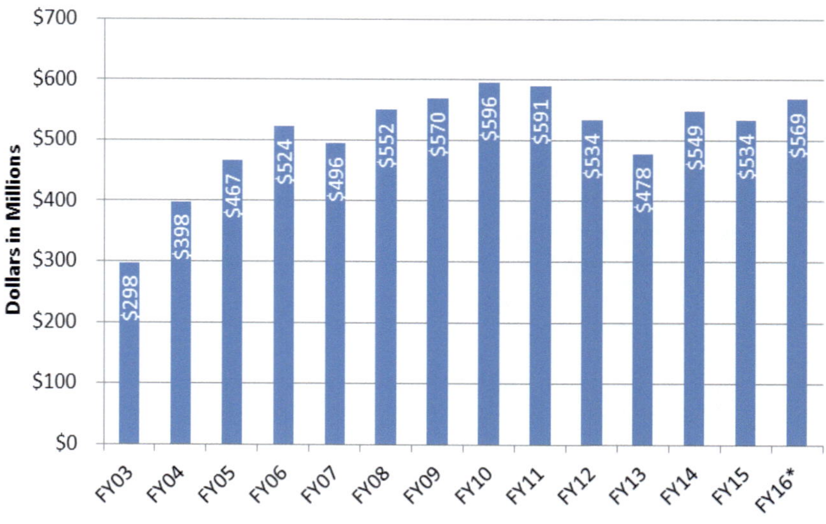


**FIGURE 3-9** Strategic National Stockpile funding history (FY 2003–FY 2016).
NOTE: *FY 16 listed at the President's Budget level, pending final appropriation.
SOURCES: Hanen presentation, March 9, 2017; from CDC.

for any state, national, or international declared public health emergency response.[15]

Lieberman outlined some of the benefits of PHEF. It can help federal, state, and local public health officials address a crisis without having to wait for Congress, so that politics do not stand in the way of the public's health. It can jump-start response efforts because money could be quickly moved to meet the immediate needs of the crisis.[16] Finally, biotechnology companies interested in researching MCMs would have some reassurance of funding stability. However, she warned that there are also potential drawbacks. Because many policy makers do not understand the distinction between preparedness and response, they may consider PHEF to be the solution to other problems, and it might be used as an excuse to cut base preparedness funding. This attitude is problematic because since FY 2005, CDC state and local preparedness funding has declined by almost one-third, and ASPR HPP funding has been cut nearly in half (see Figure 3-10).

Lieberman emphasized that funding delays have real consequences on the effectiveness of public health emergency response. Delays in distributing emergency funds not only hamper the response, but they can also stifle research and discourage involvement in the biotechnology industry. For example, one of the major consequences of the delay in the Zika virus response was that as Congress took longer and longer to appropriate money, biotechnology companies became less interested and less willing to become involved in Zika virus countermeasures research. This loss of interest hindered not only the short-term response to the Zika virus, but also long-term partnerships with those companies. She cautioned that having public–private partnerships in place in the MCM space is critically important as there is no other natural marketplace for those products, and the industry needs reassurance that the government will be a reliable partner and provide necessary funding throughout the research process. Delays in emergency funding also hurt other priorities, Lieberman noted. During PHEP reprogramming, the Zika virus response was maintained by moving $44 million from the All Hazards account. NACCHO and other organizations carried out a survey of their members to better understand

---

[15] Other proposals Lieberman and Hanen discussed included the FY 2017 House Labor–HHS CDC Infectious Disease Rapid Response Reserve Fund, which puts $300 million into CDC infectious disease rapid response (overall public health funding would also be cut, including for infectious disease); the Public Health Emergency Preparedness Act (Representative DeLauro), which would put $5 billion into PHEF; and the CDC Emergency Response Act (114th Congress) (Senator Boxer, retired), which would put $2 billion into a CDC-controlled fund.

[16] Lieberman noted that there may be many different types of public health emergencies warranting funding than are traditionally considered (e.g., the opioid epidemic; the Flint, Michigan; water crisis) that may qualify for PHEP.

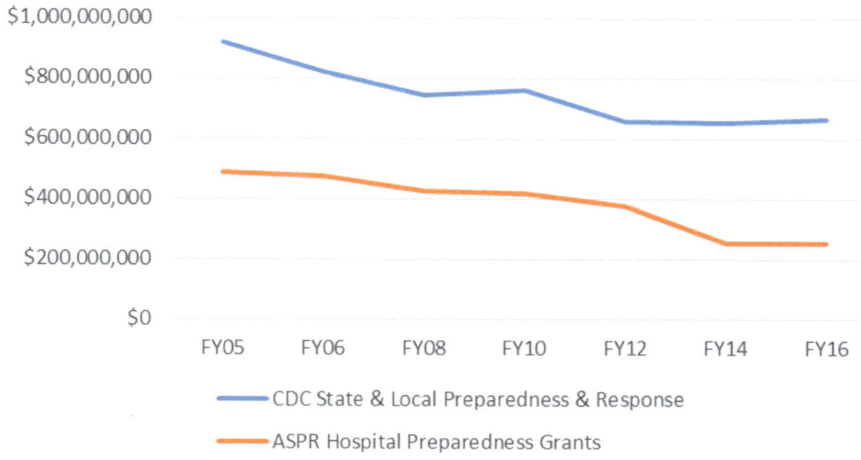


**FIGURE 3-10** CDC and ASPR preparedness funds (FY 2005–FY 2016).
NOTE: ASPR = Assistant Secretary for Preparedness and Response; CDC = U.S. Centers for Disease Control and Prevention.
SOURCE: Lieberman presentation, March 8, 2017.

the impacts of the redirected $44 million.[17] She reported that according to the survey, areas most negatively affected by PHEP funding reprogramming were pre-event readiness (74.7 percent), supplies (54.6 percent), staffing levels (47.2 percent), functional preparedness program levels (34.6 percent), and contractual services (23.5 percent). She noted that these cuts occurred in areas that could not easily be backfilled.

Lieberman stressed the importance of impressing upon policy makers that short-term, supplemental funding for a crisis cannot take the place of ongoing preparedness efforts. For example, in the years before the emergence of the Zika virus, funding for mosquito-borne surveillance was cut from $24 million to $10 million (2004–2012). A state or local health department cannot maintain a mosquito surveillance program with that type of short-term funding, she cautioned. A further concern is that the no-year fund might be viewed as an attractive funding source for Congress or HHS even with limitations incorporated into the statute to prevent another outbreak. For example, the unspent Ebola outbreak supplemental funding should have been spent on continued efforts in West Africa, but was instead

[17] See the impact of the redirection of public health emergency preparedness (PHEP) funding from state and local health departments to support national Zika response at http://www.naccho.org/uploads/downloadable-resources/Impact-of-the-Redirection-of-PHEP-Funding-to-Support-Zika-Response.pdf (accessed August 8, 2017).

shifted to the Zika virus response, and the funding for the BioShield Special Reserve Fund has instead been used for BARDA research and development.

Pressures on the discretionary budget may also lead to major cuts to public health funding, Lieberman warned. If the Patient Protection and Affordable Care Act is repealed, the repeal of the Prevention and Public Health Fund will create a nearly $1 billion shortfall in CDC's budget that will affect foundational public health capabilities in ways that short-term supplemental funding cannot cover. She stressed that PHEF can only solve the problem of delayed supplemental funding by serving as a potentially incomplete bridge between the onset of a crisis and the need for supplemental funding.[18]

Lieberman's organization recommends that PHEF require sufficient funding to bridge the gap between the onset of a crisis and the availability of supplemental funds, and that such funding must be replenished over time. She stated that moving forward will require clarifying the difference between preparedness and response for lawmakers, clarifying who is in charge between CDC and HHS, addressing bureaucratic challenges in obtaining funding, and establishing appropriate transparency and accountability to ensure that funding is being used as intended.

A critical funding challenge, Hanen argued, is that the U.S. appropriations system is broken. She explained that funding the HHS Preparedness Enterprise requires the passage of 12 spending bills. The U.S. government has been unable to pass those 12 bills in a timely fashion, which has forced a reliance on various types of short-term continuing resolutions to keep the government programs funded for a few weeks at a time.[19] She reported that 6 months into FY 2017, there still were no spending bills introduced. The uncertainty causes delays for federal agencies in their planning and spending that trickles down to both state and local health departments and ultimately creates further uncertainty for MCM developers (see Figure 3-11).

Sustained investment is critical to maintain preparedness capacity, said Hanen, but funding for public health preparedness will be affected by the overall deficit reduction debate. Although emergency funding is appreciated, a sustained investment is critical to maintain preparedness capacity in both public health and health care systems. However, due to the reduction in funding for mainstay programs, events such as an Ebola outbreak require going to Congress for emergency supplemental appropriations (e.g.,

[18] For example, Lieberman noted, if there is $1.5 billion from the Cassidy bill, but the Ebola supplement was about $5.5 billion, then Congress may use PHEF as an excuse not to provide supplemental funding in the (rare) event it is needed.

[19] Hanen discussed examples such as omnibuses that package all 12 bills together; cromnibuses (combinations of short-term continuing resolutions and other spending bills); and year-long continuing resolutions.

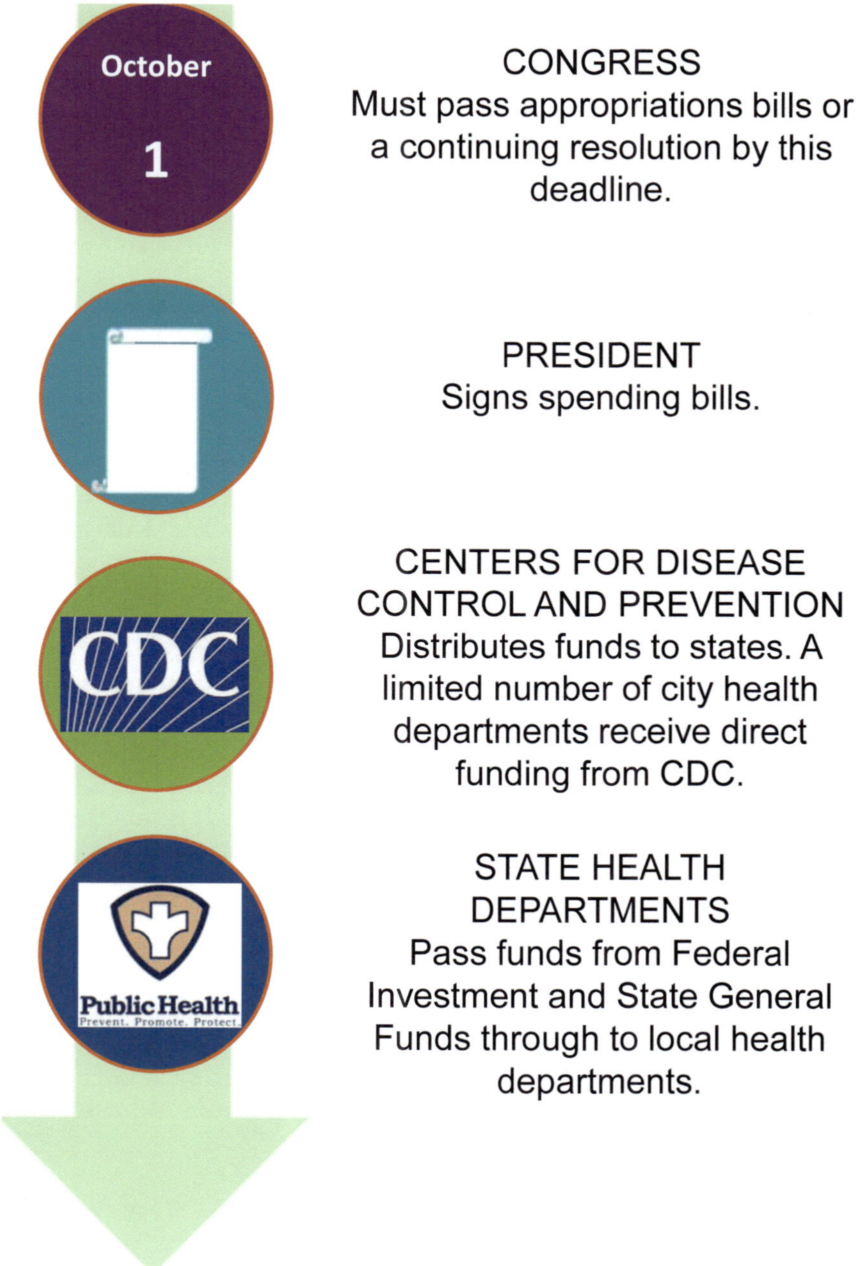


**FIGURE 3-11** Appropriations process.
SOURCE: Hanen presentation, March 9, 2017.

5-year emergency supplemental funding of $1.7 billion for Ebola outbreak, domestic, and global response, as well as GHSA). She explained that when the Zika virus outbreak occurred, Congress instructed them to dip into the approved Ebola outbreak response funding to pay for the Zika virus response, and it took Congress 7 months after the initial request to approve a Zika virus supplemental. Although the appropriators provided a 5-year appropriation for the Ebola outbreak response, the funding will likely be spent well before the 5 years is over because Congress had to dip into those resources to fund a different outbreak.

Kathryn Brinsfield, former assistant secretary of Health Affairs and chief medical officer, Office of Health Affairs, DHS, noted that public health is the prerequisite for success in health care emergency preparedness, but it requires convincing people to invest in programs that are difficult to understand. Runnels highlighted the challenge of creating a sense of urgency, particularly among decision makers who have not dealt with emergencies, to make investments and change systems at the local, state, and federal levels. Matthew Wynia, director, Center for Bioethics and Humanities, University of Colorado Denver, observed that striking the right balance of private-sector, local, and federal funding for public health preparedness is a key ongoing challenge. Richard Danila, Epidemiology Program manager and deputy state epidemiologist, Minnesota Department of Health, Council for State and Territorial Epidemiologists, noted that there are many established health care and public health infrastructure gaps and weaknesses, but correcting them requires resources that generally do not exist or will not otherwise be allocated. He stressed that more and better financial arguments and analyses will be needed to change the minds of funders and decision makers.

Shah emphasized the need to adequately fund local public health capacity first, noting that public health departments across the country are suffering because we have not invested in the systems and that local public health capacity is a critical component of on-the-ground emergency response that must be adequately funded. Onora Lien, Northwest Healthcare Response Network, noted that at the community level, the annual funding cycle and different approaches taken by various funding streams make it difficult to create alignment to mobilize all efforts toward consistent and sustained common outcomes.

## INTERSECTION BETWEEN DOMESTIC AND GLOBAL HEALTH SECURITY

Shah focused on the local perspective of how global and domestic health come together in communities. In terms of protecting the community, he likened public health to the "offensive line" (largely unknown or behind the scenes) compared with emergency medical services (EMS), fire, law enforcement, and even health care. Although it is largely invisible, he noted, public health is critical at the local community level beyond preparedness and emergency response.[20] Shah explained that economics, education, environment, and engagement, or the four "Es," are key drivers of health. He highlighted engagement as a key piece, because engaging the community requires connecting the dots between events happening across the globe and things happening rapidly in the community: "Whether it's refugee health issues, issues about unaccompanied minors, or Zika/Ebola outbreak and the like, we very quickly realize that what's happening in other parts of the globe is very much impacting our community."

According to Shah and Dan Hanfling, clinical professor, Department of Emergency Medicine, and contributing scholar, Center for Health Security, JHSPH, most Americans support international efforts to improve health in developing countries and other global settings, despite the pervasive politicization of activities and interests (see Figures 3-12 and 3-13).

Shah emphasized the ways in which global interconnectedness affects domestic communities. He noted that the impact on the United States from global events such as infectious diseases is not a new concept. For example, the HIV/AIDS epidemic started as a phenomenon that was not in local U.S. communities but moved to local communities from across the globe in the 1980s. Houston communities have a particularly bidirectional relationship with the rest of the world, he explained, because of community members who are part of the global community: it has a high degree of diversity, busy ports and airports, and a large West African community in Harris County. In the past year, his department spent $1.5 million on multidisciplinary approaches to Zika virus response. As a result of a 7-month funding delay, they were forced to repurpose physicians and other staff in order to respond to the Zika virus outbreak appropriately. Shah observed that ultimately, "The investment in what happens globally, the investment in what happens domestically, and the fact that bidirectionally you have a connection between that global and domestic health front is very much about capacity building."

Marinissen provided an overview of lessons learned from past disasters and emergencies, which spanned challenges and barriers including legal, regulatory, funding, intellectual property, logistical, information management, ethical, and U.S. government and international coordination. During H1N1 (2009), for example, there were requests for assistance from more than 50 countries; the United States deployed large amounts of H1N1

---

[20] For example, Shah noted that in Houston, community agencies spray for mosquitoes, pick up dangerous animals, conduct restaurant inspections, address foodborne illness, mitigate threats, administer vaccinations, and so forth.

vaccines and antivirals but faced enormous delays. During the Haiti earthquake (2010), despite claims that medical personnel and public health assets would never be deployed internationally due to legal, regulatory, logistical, and funding barriers, then President Obama deployed resources to Haiti and encountered many challenges. In Fukushima after the nuclear disaster (2011), there was a lack of sufficient information from modeling, discrepant messages from the U.S. government and the government of Japan, and conflicting utilization policies. During the MERS-CoV outbreak (2012), the United States needed but could not obtain samples from Saudi Arabian and South Korean labs to develop and validate diagnostic tools because there was no international consensus on terms and conditions for rapid sample sharing. During the Ebola outbreak (2013), there was a draft framework from Haiti for international deployment, but also new problems that occurred with MCMs, samples, personnel, incident command, and leadership to coordinate public health measures across borders. As a slow-moving event, the Zika virus outbreak (2015) raised the issue of how to start coordinating the research required to mount a response.

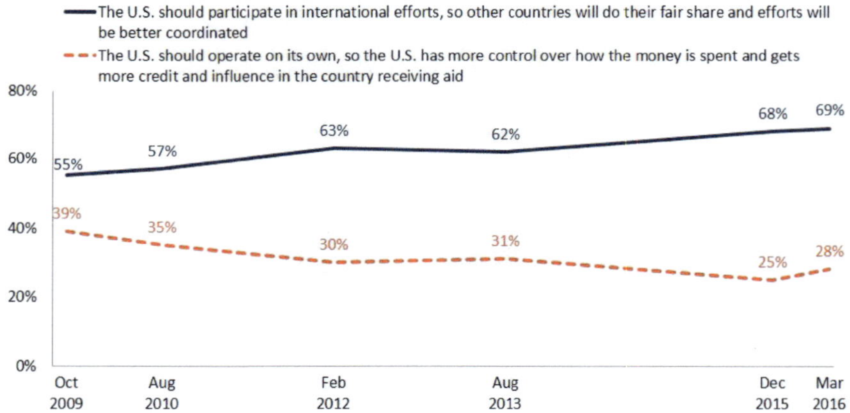


**FIGURE 3-12** Seven in 10 Americans say the United States should participate in international efforts to improve health in developing countries.
NOTE: The prompt was: Which comes closer to your opinion? When giving aid to improve health in developing countries...; Both/Neither (vol.) and Don't know/Refused responses not shown.
SOURCES: Shah presentation, March 9, 2017; Kaiser Family Foundation Surveys of Americans on the U.S. role in Global Health, Kaiser Family Foundation Health Tracking Polls.

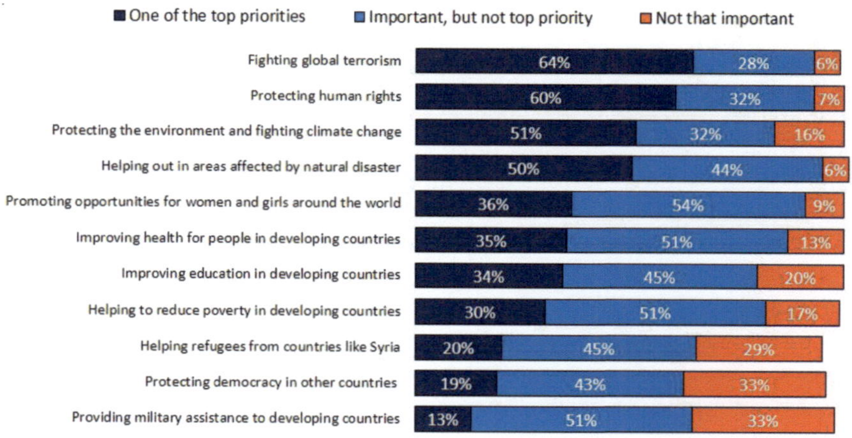


**FIGURE 3-13** Kaiser Family Foundation (2016) survey of the U.S. public about its role in international engagement.
NOTE: The prompt was: I'm going to read you some different things the president and Congress might try to do when it comes to world affairs. As I read each one, tell me if you think it should be one of their top priorities, important but not a top priority, or not that important; Some items asked of half sample. Not all important (vol.) and Don't know/Refused answers not shown.
SOURCES: Hanfling presentation, March 9, 2017; Kaiser Family Foundation 2016 Survey of Americans on the U.S. role in Global Health (conducted March 1–26, 2016).

Preparing for the next international threat requires strengthening preparedness and response at the domestic–international interface, according to Marinissen. This preparation is already under way: a global push led to the development of WHO's Health Emergencies Programme, an ASPR-like structure that brings together humanitarian system programs and the IHR community under one line of command to respond to all kinds of public health emergencies. She explained that priority areas include a unified WHO emergency program, a global health emergency workforce, IHR core capacities and resilient national health systems, improvements to IHR, accelerated research and development, and an international financing and contingency fund. The U.S. government has taken an important first step by using international standards and IHR to measure its domestic capacities via the joint external evaluation process, in which external evaluators provided useful feedback about gaps. Marinissen commended this action as representing a significant step forward in opening the doors to the international community and varying points of view.

Rebecca Katz, associate professor of International Health and co-director, Center for Global Health Science and Security, Georgetown University Medical Center, focused on the challenge of sustaining a commitment to GHSA and its consequences for the future of global health security. She sketched the evolution of GHSA, explaining that the topic was raised in earnest on the political agenda in 2011, when President Obama stated in a speech at the United Nations General Assembly: "We must come together to prevent, detect, and fight every kind of biological danger—whether it's a pandemic like H1N1, or a terrorist threat, or a treatable disease" (September 22, 2011). This speech, and the momentum behind it, prompted what would eventually become GHSA, which was launched in early 2014 by the United States, 28 other national governments, and 3 international organizations. It is now a partnership of more than 55 countries, with the intent to accelerate progress toward preparing the world for biological threats. She explained that some of these countries are donor states and some play more of a recipient role, but the goal is to come together and contribute to shaping the agenda. The agenda is shaped in part by being organized around capacity building for prevention, detection, and response through 11 action packages with specific targets and metrics according to which countries develop best practices and focus their investments.[21]

Katz underscored some of the successes already achieved pertaining to GHSA, which has employed the strategy of raising political awareness to mitigate threat. The first success has been marshalling resources, she noted. The United States had a one-time appropriation of $1 billion focused on a set of priority countries; Korea committed to provide $100 million to focus on 13 different countries. The G7 made a commitment to support 76 countries with an undetermined amount of money. Political recognition and coordination have made global health security and response to biological threats part of discussions with heads of states. Through forums such as G20, a series of GHSA high-level ministerial meetings, world leaders are actively discussing the best pathways for reducing biological threats. By marshaling these resources, GHSA has helped to build a national capacity to rapidly detect and respond to biological events. She argued that this rapid detection and response capacity directly translates into being able to save lives in the event of a public health emergency (see Figure 3-14).

Katz continued that the GHSA has spurred the international community to accept external evaluations of national capacities for prevention, detection, and response. The joint external evaluation tool is now being used in conjunction with the IHR; 29 have been completed so far, 31 more

[21] Katz further explained that GHSA action packages include antimicrobial resistance, zoonotic disease, biosafety and biosecurity, immunization, national laboratory systems, real-time surveillance, reporting, workforce development, emergency operations centers, linking public health with law and multisectoral rapid response, MCMs, and personnel deployment.

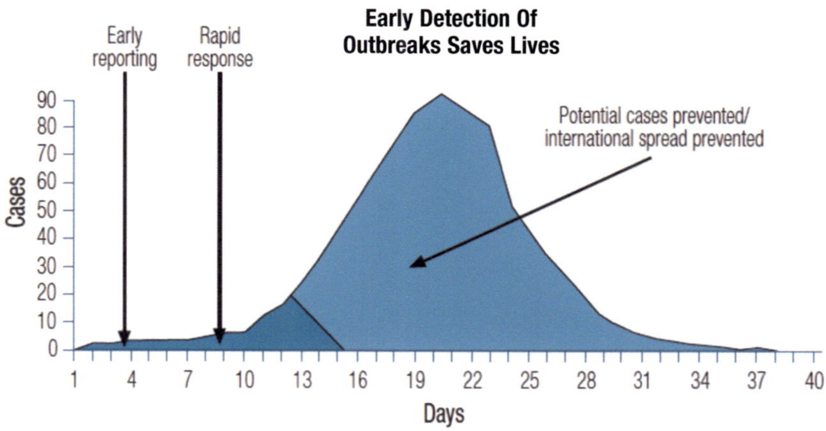


**FIGURE 3-14** Early detection of outbreaks.
SOURCES: Katz presentation, March 9, 2017; The world health report 2007-Global Public Health Security in the 21st Century. A safer future, http://www.who.int/whr/2007/whr07_en.pdf (accessed January 10, 2018). Figure 2 Global outbreaks, the challenge: late reporting.

are in the pipeline, and an additional 27 countries have expressed interest, she reported (see Figure 3-15).

At the February 2017 Munich Security Summit, Hanfling reported, Bill Gates emphasized the issue of biosecurity and the tremendous risk at hand: "A fast-moving airborne pathogen could kill more than 30 million people in less than a year." Katz presented an overview of the threat of infectious disease over the past 60 years, during which time the number of new diseases per decade has quadrupled. The number of outbreaks per year has tripled since 1980, with the majority being zoonotic in origin.[22]

Katz explained that if a disease emerges in one part of the world, it can be anywhere else within 24 to 48 hours due to globalization and the movement of people, animals, and goods. Recent examples of emerging infectious diseases over the past decade include the severe acute respiratory syndrome outbreak in South China; MERS-CoV in Saudi Arabia and South Korea; the Ebola outbreak in West Africa; Zika virus in the Americas; the resurgence of polio, particularly in fragile states; the more recent outbreaks of yellow fever; and the ever-present threat of new variants of influenza. She clarified that the threat is not only one of naturally occurring disease,

---

[22] See http://www.npr.org/sections/goatsandsoda/2017/02/07/512634375/map-find-out-what-new-viruses-are-emerging-in-your-backyard (accessed September 19, 2017).

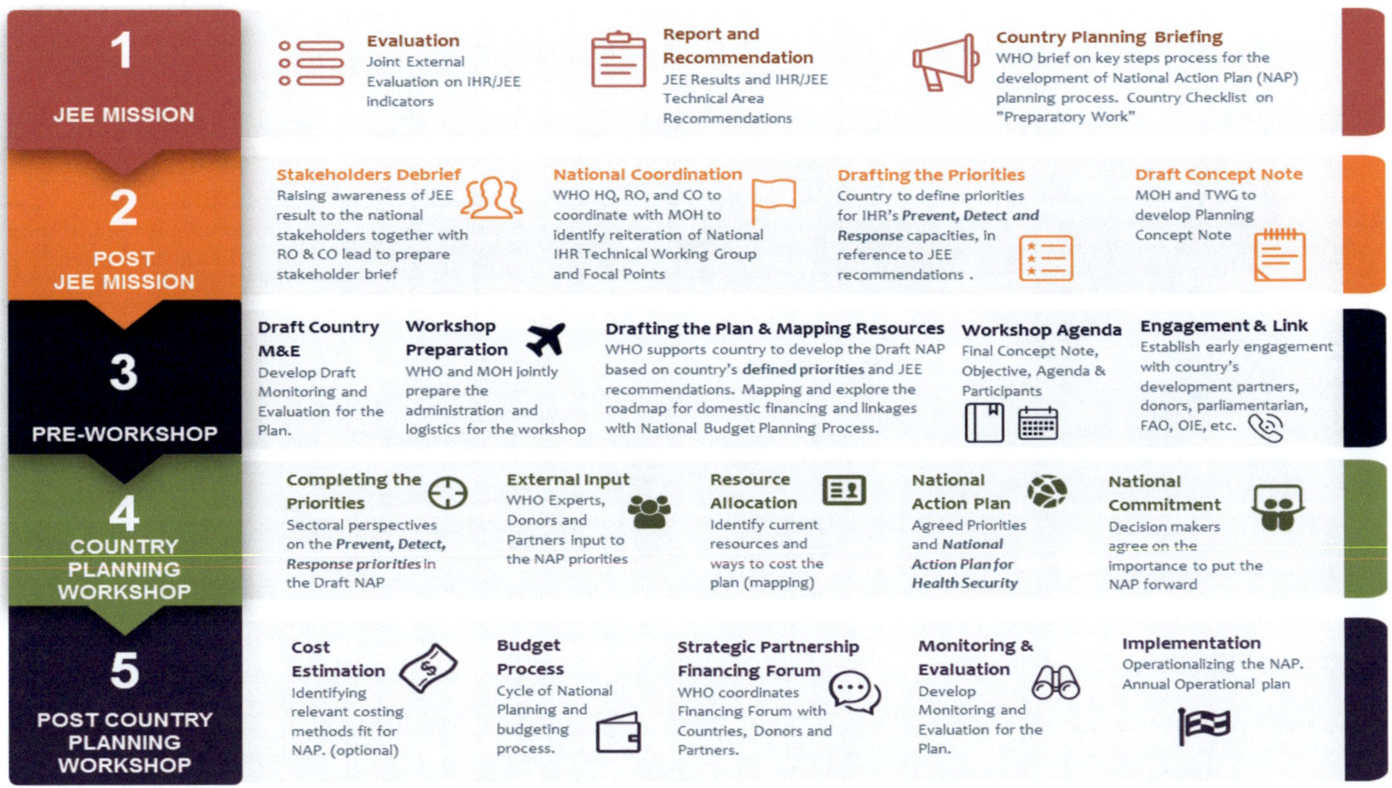
1
JEE MISSION
Evaluation
Joint External Evaluation on IHR/JEE indicators
Report and Recommendation
JEE Results and IHR/JEE Technical Area Recommendations
Country Planning Briefing
WHO brief on key steps process for the development of National Action Plan (NAP) planning process. Country Checklist on "Preparatory Work"
2
POST JEE MISSION
Stakeholders Debrief
Raising awareness of JEE result to the national stakeholders together with RO & CO lead to prepare stakeholder brief
National Coordination
WHO HQ, RO, and CO to coordinate with MOH to identify reiteration of National IHR Technical Working Group and Focal Points
Drafting the Priorities
Country to define priorities for IHR's Prevent, Detect and Response capacities, in reference to JEE recommendations .
Draft Concept Note
MOH and TWG to develop Planning Concept Note
3
PRE-WORKSHOP
Draft Country M&E
Develop Draft Monitoring and Evaluation for the Plan.
Workshop Preparation
WHO and MOH jointly prepare the administration and logistics for the workshop
Drafting the Plan & Mapping Resources
WHO supports country to develop the Draft NAP based on country's defined priorities and JEE recommendations. Mapping and explore the roadmap for domestic financing and linkages with National Budget Planning Process.
Workshop Agenda
Final Concept Note, Objective, Agenda & Participants
Engagement & Link
Establish early engagement with country's development partners, donors, parliamentarian, FAO, OIE, etc.
4
COUNTRY PLANNING WORKSHOP
Completing the Priorities
Sectoral perspectives on the Prevent, Detect, Response priorities in the Draft NAP
External Input
WHO Experts, Donors and Partners input to the NAP priorities
Resource Allocation
Identify current resources and ways to cost the plan (mapping)
National Action Plan
Agreed Priorities and National Action Plan for Health Security
National Commitment
Decision makers agree on the importance to put the NAP forward
5
POST COUNTRY PLANNING WORKSHOP
Cost Estimation
Identifying relevant costing methods fit for NAP. (optional)
Budget Process
Cycle of National Planning and budgeting process.
Strategic Partnership Financing Forum
WHO coordinates Financing Forum with Countries, Donors and Partners.
Monitoring & Evaluation
Develop Monitoring and Evaluation for the Plan.
Implementation
Operationalizing the NAP. Annual Operational plan

**FIGURE 3-15** GHSA joint external evaluations.

NOTE: CO = Country Office; FAO = Food and Agriculture Organization; GHSA = Global Health Security Agenda; HO = home office; IHR = International Health Regulations; JEE = Joint External Evaluation; MoH = Ministry of Health; OIE = World Organisation for Animal Health; RO = Regional Office; TWG = Technical Working Group; WHO = World Health Organization.

SOURCES: Katz presentation, March 9, 2017; reprinted from Update on JEE and Country Planning Post JEE-GHSA Steering Group Meeting, 21 January 2017, see https://www.ghsagenda.org/docs/default-source/default-document-library/jee-and-country-planning-post-jee-508.pdf (accessed October 2, 2017).

but also of the ever-present danger of a deliberate event that could have massive consequences. She explained that models demonstrate that such events are possible and maybe even probable within the next 15 years. Modelers also expect a large-scale pandemic every 100 to 150 years, and the 100th anniversary of the 1918 influenza epidemic is approaching. Aside from large-scale potential events, on a day-to-day basis there are biological threats emerging around the world that require functional public health infrastructure to address them. She noted that last year alone, WHO received more than 60,000 reports of biological events, 300 disease alerts identified for follow-up every month, and more than one field investigation carried out each day.

Katz cautioned about the current lack of global preparedness: "There is a very real need for public health infrastructure, but we are unprepared even with the known threat." She explained that IHR obligates countries to develop certain core capacities to detect, assess, report, and respond to public health emergencies. However, she reported that as of 2012, only 22 percent of countries had fully developed this capacity and by 2014, only 33 percent of countries had (see Figure 3-16).

Several workshop participants further examined the challenges faced in strengthening U.S. efforts in international public health disaster emergency response, as well as sustaining the commitment to GHSA. Hanfling, a practicing emergency physician with 20 years of urban search and rescue response experience with the U.S. Agency for International Development (USAID) and FEMA, focused on the critical challenge of coordinating domestic and international emergency response. International disaster response is critically important, emphasized Hanfling: "Despite the milieu in which the discussions occur, we know that delayed response costs lives." He noted that during World War II, President Roosevelt entered the war only after the attack on Pearl Harbor, at which point millions of lives had already been lost in Europe. Hanfling cited the Ebola outbreak as a recent example of the impact of delay on the ability to galvanize resources, brain power, and expertise that the United States can bring to these discussions.

Marinissen highlighted the challenge of working with U.S. and international partners to strengthen public health preparedness and response at the domestic–international interface: not by working only on domestic preparedness or on international preparedness, but by working on those two together in an integrated way. She explained this coordination will require public health and health systems capacity building around the world and in the United States, as well as preparedness and response planning to enable response with the international community. Regarding FEMA's National Response Framework[23] for how the government organizes itself

[23] See https://www.fema.gov/national-response-framework (accessed August 8, 2017).

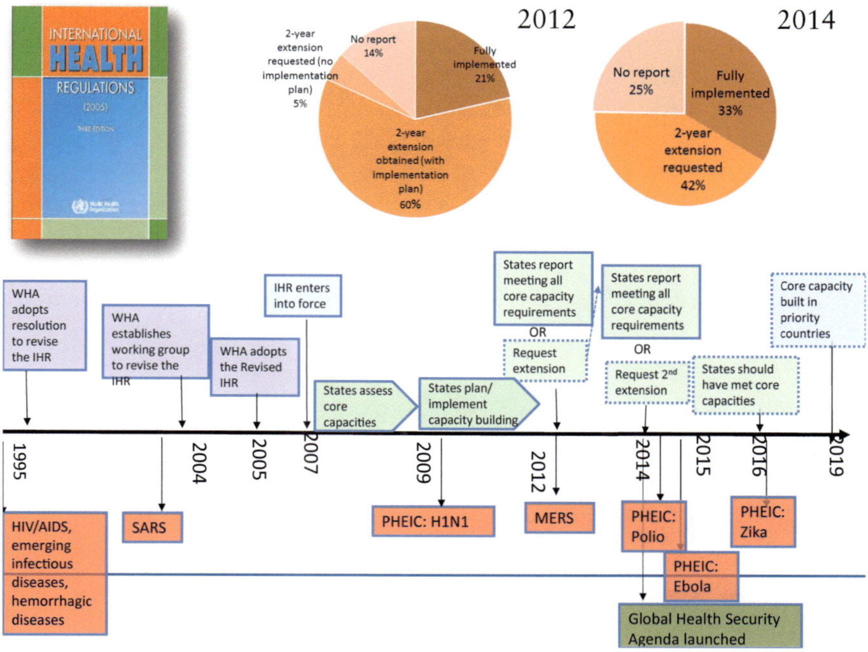


**FIGURE 3-16** IHR compliance.
NOTE: HIV/AIDS = human immunodeficiency virus/acquired immunodeficiency syndrome; IHR = International Health Regulations; MERS = Middle East respiratory syndrome; PHEIC = public health emergency of international concern; SARS = severe acute respiratory syndrome; WHA = World Health Assembly.
SOURCE: Katz presentation, March 9, 2017.

and integrates community assistance to respond to terrorist attacks, natural disasters, and other catastrophic events, Marinissen noted that international coordination (Annex-Emergency Support Function #8) is still unclear. The U.S. Department of State is briefly discussed as being the lead; however, there is no indication of how it interacts with other agencies, such as HHS and USAID. Kurilla noted that broad processes are in place internationally that are not specific to a particular emerging infectious disease or public health outbreak response. Review processes, cycle times, funding decisions, and so forth are not aligned across different countries, which is an issue that cannot be effectively addressed in the midst of a crisis, when consensus is impossible to reach.

Katz also outlined a set of challenges related to strengthening the U.S. commitment to GHSA. The first pertains to funding: the United States provided a one-time appropriation, but it is not clear if funding will be continued. Even though GHSA is designed to help coordinate efforts, there are cases of multiple countries funding a single action package in one country, while other countries are neglected. Another challenge relates to where resources are invested, she remarked. The countries receiving capacity-building assistance are not necessarily the same countries or regions that are the most likely to experience an emerging infectious disease, according to hotspot analyses. On the political side, she noted, GHSA is an initiative of the Obama administration. Without knowing the intent of the Trump administration, with some notable exceptions like the President's Emergency Plan for AIDS Relief, initiatives that are closely associated with a previous administration are not always necessarily championed by the new administration.

## VULNERABLE POPULATIONS AND COMMUNITY RESILIENCE

David Eisenman, director, Fielding School of Public Health, University of California, Los Angeles, defined community resilience as the capacity of the community as a whole to prepare for, respond to, and recover from adverse events. According to theory and research, he explained, strong social and organizational networks are critical for improving resilience, as are examining and strengthening existing resources. He outlined a set of challenges in communicating, training, and scaling community resilience programs. There is often a cultural disconnect between two "tribes": resilience coalitions that adhere to a collective action and empowerment approach in which the process is paramount, and emergency public health nurses and first responders who feel knowledgeable going into a response but have also witnessed failures of that process first hand. He suggested that if resilience is to be focused on bringing diverse sectors together for collective action, then the public health workforce must be better trained for future responses. Furthermore, he noted that resilience will require public health to find new ways to bring diverse sectors together toward collective action and planning. Another question going forward is whether public health departments can, or will, use a scalable model of community resilience programs that is embedded in the ongoing work in chronic disease, violence prevention, and other areas of day-to-day focus.

Communities directly affected by disasters are not the only ones that benefit from resilience. Redlener highlighted the destination communities that receive evacuees as a neglected dimension: "There is not a single hamlet, town, or city in America that is adequately prepared to deal with the displaced people over a long period of time. They need jobs . . . health care . . . food and water . . . schools. What is happening to the economy in a place where they left and the place to where they are going?" Redlener explained that the experience of evacuation can also be traumatic. He described the logistics of evacuation, especially during the type of spontaneous and chaotic evacuation that may occur after a mega-disaster, as "horrendous and overwhelmingly challenging." For example, many people will evacuate in private vehicles, and people will need to be picked up from within contaminated areas; displaced people must remain where they go for a long period of time. Redlener offered a health care and public health perspective on some of the many challenges faced by evacuees and destination communities:

- Separation from loved ones and dependents;
- Psychological concerns, such as extreme return uncertainty and the end of normalcy;
- Loss of possessions;
- Loss of pets;
- Injuries, such as blunt trauma, radiation, burns, and shock;
- Hunger and thirst;
- Acute evacuation trauma, such as motor vehicle accidents;
- Acute illness, such as myocardial infarction, cerebral vascular accident, and acute respiratory problems;
- Complications of chronic disease: diabetic ketoacidosis, severe hypertension;
- Loss of medication (and critical device) access; and
- Feeling disoriented and terrified.

Vulnerable populations need special, focused attention during a disaster, Redlener explained, characterizing this challenge as the Achilles' heel(s) of disaster response. He estimated that between one-third to one-half of the U.S. population has some sort of disability. Dan Dodgen, director, Division for At-Risk Individuals, Behavioral Health, and Community Resilience, ASPR, HHS, suggested that to improve individual- and community-level preparedness, the focus should be placed on the people most at risk (although that group can be difficult to define). However, there is an evidential basis for groups most at risk (Brunkard et al., 2008; WHO, 2011; World Bank, 2013). Worldwide, 30 to 50 percent of disaster fatalities are children. During Hurricane Katrina, 50 percent of fatalities were over the age of 75. Women comprised 70 percent of the casualties in the 2004 Indian Ocean tsunami.

Abramson described the community system of Gerritsen Beach in Brooklyn, a middle-class neighborhood home to multigenerational families. Most homes sustained major to moderate damage as a result of Hurricane Sandy, and the community was comprehensively damaged. Residents were accustomed to dealing with their own problems and were unprepared for a situation in which an emergency struck all of them at once, leaving them unable to rely on each other. This situation caused increases in mental health distress and alcoholism, among other consequences. Abramson reflected that "essentially, their problems eluded the systems above them. Nobody was able to see their problems." He explained how the California wildfires (2007–2008) raised the issue of undocumented immigrants who would not evacuate because they were concerned about losing their jobs or being deported from the United States. Recognition of this problem led to a rapid research CDC grant to identify issues among undocumented immigrants in four cities within 2 months of the H1N1 outbreak. It emerged that the undocumented immigrants were relying on community-based organizations in their communities to help them mediate and broker information. These community-based organizations serving as trusted information brokers were critical to the more isolated or vulnerable communities of undocumented immigrants, he reported. This research also revealed a willingness by undocumented immigrants to engage with certain trusted public officials, particularly around health issues (U.S. physicians and public health officials were particularly trusted).

Abramson summarized findings and lessons learned from a set of tabletop exercises on reaching specific at-risk populations and potentially elusive groups (e.g., urban teens, rural homebound people and their caregivers, people living with HIV, and undocumented Latin American immigrants). Living lab scenarios[24] were designed to examine engagement strategies, needs and wants, trusted allies, and potential issues for each elusive group. The exercise revealed that messaging could lead to elusive groups feeling stigmatized. For example, groups with mobility (homebound) or transportation access issues are sensitive to messages that imply an allocation of a scarce resource (i.e., "last in line" syndrome). Groups with stigma or issues regarding disclosure about their condition tend to be sensitive to messages that imply eligibility criteria or patient identification requirements. Abramson stressed that "households are as prepared or as resilient as their weakest and most vulnerable member." Furthermore, he noted, the exercise revealed that teenagers wanted to be involved and could function as critical fulcrums for families by providing translation, access to new technologies, and information sources. This unanticipated peer influence led to enhanced preparedness. Abramson suggested there could be a useful role for community-based tabletops as a preparedness intervention, and Redlener suggested ways communities might become better prepared to accept individuals who have been forced to evacuate (see Box 3-1).

[24] Abramson discussed three scenarios. Scenario 1: a pandemic outbreak with message directing the population to community-based points of dispensation (subthemes: stigma, disclosure, access); Scenario 2: a toxic gas release with message directing the population to evacuate and register with family reunification systems (subthemes: disclosure, transportation and mobility, trust); Scenario 3: an Ebola-like viral outbreak with message directing the population to isolate and quarantine (subthemes: risk uncertainty, trust, preparedness, informal supports).

**BOX 3-1**
**Evacuations: Suggested To-Do List for Host Communities**

Redlener noted that destination communities for mass evacuations are an often-overlooked dimension in preparedness and response. He suggested the following "to-do" list for host communities:

- Shelter
- Sanitation
- Reliable supply chains: food, water, medicines, diapers, cribs
- Communications and messaging
- Public safety
- Reunification
- Medical care: acute, chronic, mental health support, in-patient care
- Educational continuity and day care
- Permanent housing
- Economic opportunities
- Language and cultural accommodations
- Special populations: prisoners, nursing home residents

SOURCE: Redlener presentation, March 8, 2017.

Inglesby raised the issue of carrying out preparedness and community resilience work in the environment created around immigrants and refugees in the United States in early 2017, given the reactions to proposed or enacted immigration and security policies. Hanfling called these policies a retrograde step that may force the immigrant community back underground, where they will not seek help in anything other than life-or-death situations. He stressed that these groups—who are not just vulnerable, but disenfranchised—have been put on notice and are at great risk: "I think it is going to be incumbent on us to make sure that we figure out how to reach out and make sure that we have connections into those communities." Eisenman observed that public health is often perceived as the most trusted agency in government, but most people cannot define public health in practice because "government is government" and the distinction between government and public health is an academic one for most people: "As long as there are problems with trust in government, there will be problems with trust in public health."

Wynia pointed to the challenge of communicating information to the public about threat, risk, and vulnerability in a compelling way that is neither alarmist nor runs the risk of being dismissed. Alson suggested that the public is tired of hearing "the sky is falling" messaging about potential disasters that do not actually happen. Abramson warned that city officials often use risk communication as a directive rather than an invitation to a dialogue (e.g., "we will get in touch with you when we need to"). Elise Rowe, ASPR, HHS, highlighted the challenge of combatting negative public perceptions and disenfranchisement with the research community, the preparedness community, and academia.

Hick characterized the current messaging to the public as misleading and offering false assurances about the actual level of preparedness. He argued that the public needs clear messaging to understand the consequences of scaled-back services and the definite and palpable risk of not having response capabilities and systems in place when an incident occurs: "We must radically alter the conversation if we really want to do anything about the problems."

Alleyne noted the challenge of more effectively translating data for the public to improve the public interface with information. He related an example, from the local health department perspective, of communicating the risks associated with cancer in a community where people were convinced there was a cluster (despite no evidential link) and perceived the government as trying to hide the existence of cancer clusters across the country. He also raised the related issue of how to reach the public with accurate information given the large amount of false and/or misleading information that is circulated. Abramson commented on the powerful role of community systems in shaping everyday lives. There is no single incident commander in a community's network of systems, but there are many institutions involved: faith communities, civic and fraternal organizations, volunteer fire houses, families, and so forth. He noted that within this network, information passes informally and is richly contextualized by the specific community. Abramson outlined a set of challenges faced by the health and human services systems affecting their ability to respond to community needs: "Can they get there? Do they know where their clients are? Do they know what people need? Is there an effective incident command system [ICS] for health service, and can it acquire the information it needs to 'direct' the system?"

Dodgen also commented on the challenge of better integrating the perspectives and needs of the community into emergency response because investment in public engagement activities has had little effect on individual- or community-level preparedness. Dodgen attributed this in part to ongoing challenges of how to successfully engage the entire community, deciding who to bring to the table (e.g., seniors, children, people with disabilities), and how to integrate all perspectives. Mandates, directives, and guidance are confusing and at times conflicting. Various organizations use different terminology to define subpopulations,[25] Dodgen explained, and even defining the concept of a community is challenging. He suggested using a common-sense rule to guide the definition of communities, goods, services, producers, consumers, and community helpers. According to Dodgen, the consequences of failure to integrate the community perspective and needs are lawsuits, bad publicity, and "failing to do our jobs." However, the consequences of success are resilient, prepared communities and positive health outcomes after a disaster.

[25] For instance, Dodgen gave the following examples of differing terminology. ASPR uses the phrase *at-risk individuals*; CDC tends to prefer *vulnerable populations* because it thinks in terms of disease risk; and FEMA has two competing favorite terminologies: *whole community* and *access and functional needs*.

# 4

# Underlying Issues in Health Security

Challenges can hinder all facets of the tightly interrelated and co-dependent health care and public health sector, and a lack of resilience in one part places an added burden on the sector as a whole. The following sections examine the participants' discussions about an overarching set of issues that pervade the sphere of health security, from an overreliance on response strategies to a lack of understanding and awareness by those with authority. Understanding the challenges can enhance the health care and public health sector's ability to prepare, respond, and recover.

## ADAPTIVE AND TECHNICAL CHALLENGES

Runnels drew a distinction between the adaptive and technical aspects of such challenges. Challenges that are more technical in nature tend to have problems and solutions that are relatively clear and easily defined; the path from point A to point B is understood, albeit not necessarily easy to traverse. She explained that adaptive issues may be difficult to define and have solutions that are not necessarily clear; the path from point A to point B is uncertain. Adaptive challenges often emerge from stakeholders' values, loyalties, and what they stand to lose if the status quo changes. Runnels reflected: "What if the adaptive problem is stemming from ourselves as a group? What can we do to challenge our deeply rooted beliefs? We are really comfortable being the solution finders and putting out fires, but maybe that is not the best place to spend our energy."

## MULTIPLE AND COMPLEX SYSTEMS

Abramson explained that every disaster response involves the activation of several complex systems: emergency management and response systems, health and human services systems, and community and kinship systems. Each of those systems has its own rules, its own structures, and its own dynamics. Figure 4-1 illustrates the complexity of the network of systems activated during the September 11, 2001, emergency response.

Abramson explained that within each of these three systems, there are variable degrees of two integral components: structured information and community context. The emergency management and response systems have the most structured information and the least amount of community context, while the community and kinship systems have the least amount of structured information and the greatest amount of community context. He described the health and human services systems as falling somewhere in the middle, but the dynamics within this system are often unclear. He illustrated this point with the example of New York City after Hurricane Sandy. Hospitals transferred particular patient populations into the communities, which created a surge for the home health and visiting nurse systems. As a result, other patients with complex treatment regimens (e.g., renal dialysis, HIV/AIDS, end-stage renal disease, methadone maintenance treatment programs) could no longer access their ambulatory care clinics. He highlighted the "last mile" problem of connecting and integrating the emergency system, the health and human services system, and the community and kinship system as a critical challenge going forward.

Kurilla also commented on the adaptive nature of integrating an entirely new conceptual strategy for approaching a problem into these existing systems (i.e., changing the rules) when the status quo is to focus on incremental change toward faster and less expensive solutions. During a response, "usually in the midst of a crisis, we'll pay for it, but in the absence of a crisis, usually the cheaper has to dominate, and so we sort of shortchange that intercrisis period, which hobbles our ability to be prepared."

According to Kurilla, finding ways to coordinate and collaborate effectively with sectors of government that may not have emergency response in their bailiwick can be problematic when such sectors are given a very specific task that is independent of the need to either be fast or slow depending on the external situation, because from their perspectives, the requirements and expectations do not change. To illustrate, he explained that the mission of human resources is specifically to maintain and ensure the integrity of the hiring process. If there are any irregularities, human resources will be blamed, but if there are no irregularities, they get no credit. If Congress provides a large supplement to address a problem, and a wide array of contract actions must be instituted but a future investigation reveals a minor

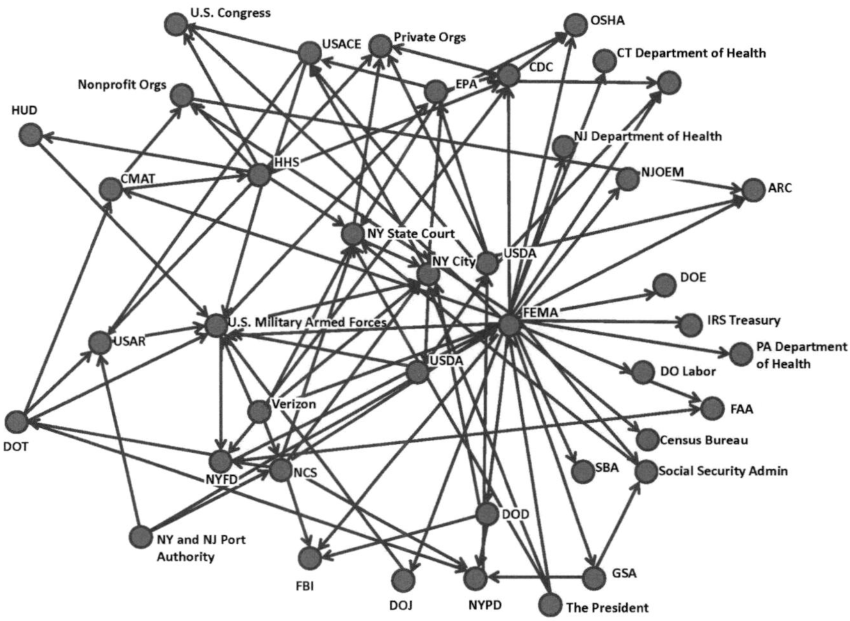


**FIGURE 4-1** Network of emergency requests from one entity to another on September 11, 2001.
NOTES: Based on FEMA situation report requests during September 11, 2001, response. ARC = American Red Cross; CDC = U.S. Centers for Disease Control and Prevention; CMAT = Crash Mapping Analysis Tool; CT = Connecticut; DO Labor = U.S. Department of Labor; DOD = U.S. Department of Defense; DOE = U.S. Department of Energy; DOJ = U.S. Department of Justice; DOT = U.S. Department of Transportation; EPA = U.S. Environmental Protection Agency; FAA = Federal Aviation Administration; FBI = Federal Bureau of Investigation; FEMA = Federal Emergency Management Agency; GSA = General Services Administration; HHS = U.S. Department of Health and Human Services; HUD = U.S. Department of Housing and Urban Development; IRS = Internal Revenue Service; NCS = National ComNet Services; NJ = New Jersey; NJOEM = New Jersey Office of Emergency Management; NY = New York; NYFD = New York Fire Department; NYPD = New York Police Department; OSHA = Occupational Safety and Health Administration; PA = Pennsylvania; SBA = U.S. Small Business Administration; USACE = U.S. Army Corps of Engineers; USAR = U.S. Army Reserve; USDA = U.S. Department of Agriculture.
SOURCES: Abramson presentation, March 8, 2017; Kapucu, 2005.

irregularity, those in charge of the contracts will be called to task despite being pushed by outside forces to institute the contracts quickly. Kurilla reported that he has put recent efforts into arguing that preparedness should be considered a bona fide need that is the criteria for justifying contracts.

## COMPETING PRIORITIES AND PERCEPTIONS

Lori Peek, author, *Children of Katrina*, and director, Natural Hazards Center and Professor of Sociology, University of Colorado, discussed the challenge of incentivizing problem solving for issues such as critical infrastructure protection between disasters. Hanfling reflected that this issue might be due to the competing calculus for identifying priorities in critical infrastructure protection: an emergency manager may think about critical infrastructure protection as strengthening buildings and hard space, while an emergency physician may think about it as breaking down those walls to provide access to care. Hanfling suggested that the challenge is brokering that calculus between many competing priorities. Andrew Pavia, University of Utah, also highlighted the absence of a system for prioritizing and coordinating infrastructure protection efforts. For example, in some areas community hospitals would likely bear the brunt of maintaining critical infrastructure in a disaster, but they have not invested in preparing because they do not perceive themselves as indispensable like larger hub facilities that have made investments in protection. Hick commented that getting communities to value critical infrastructure protection will be important in addressing this challenge and incentivizing interim preparation.

Abramson cautioned that other sectors may erroneously perceive the public good as a zero-sum game, giving rise to collaboration problems. For example, he noted that the 58 city hospitals in New York City have competing interests that engender unwillingness and tension in trying to collaborate. Alson noted that state- and local-level agencies have their own sets of competing priorities that often are their first concern and obfuscate the broader picture of what needs to be achieved.

## DIFFICULTY DEFINING GOALS AND INTERPRETING PROGRESS

Redlener identified the "denominator problem" as determining what is needed versus what has been done. He suggested that if preparedness is a spectrum between 0 percent prepared (the starting state) to 100 percent prepared (which is impossible), within that spectrum falls both the current state of readiness and an ideal realistic state of readiness, with the latter determined by the local context for defining preparedness. The challenge is how to interpret the change (delta) between the starting state and the current state. The typical interpretation—"we are doing fine because we're making progress"—is much more problematic, he argued, than the interpretation that things are behind where they ought to be: "We must understand where we are going, how we are going to get there, and be honest about where we are."

Measures of success also vary across sectors, remarked Brinsfield. Other sectors measure success objectively (e.g., what can be produced). Public health and health care, she noted, tend to measure success by "whether we are doing the most we can with the money we have, or whether we are successfully moving forward," rather than objectively assessing the potential outcomes of different available strategies prior to implementing a plan of action.

## LACK OF RESOURCES TO SUPPORT DATA-DRIVEN IMPROVEMENT

Runnels noted that people respond reactively to many disasters and questioned why there is a lack of upfront investment in preparedness and resilience. Hick highlighted two fundamental reasons for critical infrastructure protection: cost and time. Identifying the deficits requires a dedicated analysis of all components that contribute to the whole. Once the deficits are identified, Hick noted that a compelling case must be built to convince an institution to address them (especially in an older institution that requires costly retrofits), with clear arguments to establish the cost of inaction for employee safety, patient safety, public safety, and the economy.

As Wolf noted, the threat to a community is constantly evolving during an emergency, which gives rise to many challenges about how to collect, validate, and disseminate data on risk and threat information, as well as prioritizing and measuring mitigation efforts. Margaret L. Brandeau, professor of management science and engineering and medicine, Stanford University, explained that processing risk and threat information requires gathering information from multiple sources, determining the risk and level of uncertainty, and then disseminating information about risks and actions that can be taken to mitigate risk. Brinsfield suggested that the challenge will be developing a true understanding of how to carry out meaningful, continually updated risk and threat assessments in the bio space. W. Craig Vanderwagen, co-founder and director, East West Protection, LLC, also noted the ongoing challenge of understanding and mitigating not only hazards, but vulnerabilities.

## OVERRELIANCE ON RESPONSE STRATEGIES

Kurilla pointed out that a clear-cut distinction between response and preparedness is not often well articulated by practitioners. As a result, the development of the field has focused primarily on response and less so on preparedness, even though, as Brinsfield emphasized, prevention is the ultimate public health preparedness. According to Sally Phillips, deputy assistant secretary for policy, ASPR, HHS, the disproportionate focus on response was born of necessity. She remarked that the lack of an evidence base makes it difficult to disseminate and integrate response and preparedness into proactive policy and planning. Redlener further commented that preparedness is context specific, meaning different things for a city, hospital, health system, or a nation. Therefore, Redlener noted, a foundational gap, particularly for governments, is precisely defining preparedness in order to establish goals, benchmarks, and budgets.

This disconnect exists in part because of the firm belief in the field that each disaster or public health emergency is unique, even though emergencies and disasters are often subsumed under the same category, as noted by Stephen C. Redd, rear admiral, U.S. Public Health Service, and director, Office of Public Health Preparedness and Response, CDC, HHS. Brandeau explained how the characteristics of disasters vary widely along multiple dimensions. Timelines for emergencies can range from hours or days (e.g., an explosion in a fertilizer plant) to weeks or months (e.g., an Anthrax letter) to months or years (e.g., Zika virus). The level of uncertainty varies as well, she noted. For example, in the case of Hurricane Katrina, the appropriate response to people's needs was fairly well understood, but the Ebola outbreak presented much more uncertainty. The affected population may vary from specific people (e.g., in a flood) to specific groups (e.g., pregnant women for the Zika virus) to everyone (e.g., some sort of infectious disease outbreak). She also explained that during any public health emergency, information develops over time, in different places, and comes from different domestic and international sources (e.g., CDC, state, county, city, public health departments, and clinicians).

Redd commented that different emergencies require different types of preparation—a natural weather disaster versus the Zika virus outbreak, for example—although the structures for those responses might be similar. Although some fundamental capabilities are already in place, Redd remarked that there is still much work to be done to prepare for different categories of emergencies. He described three broad categories: predictable emergencies that will definitely happen (e.g., hurricanes and earthquakes), predicted emergencies of high consequence that may never happen (e.g., anthrax attack) but require "very exquisite readiness to be able to respond almost instantaneously," and emerging events (e.g., Ebola and Zika virus outbreaks).

Several attendees provided examples of how current policies, rules, and guidance do not support the behaviors and practices needed to improve health care and public health preparedness, response, and recovery. Hick commented that there is an existing wealth of information in the public sector from regulatory and standards organizations relating to continuity of operations and critical infrastructure protection;[1] however, they lack sufficient specificity. Hick argued that these requirements are completely inadequate to enable facilities to appropriately mitigate risk. To illustrate, he quoted the entirety of the language from the National Fire Protection Association's *Standard on Disaster/Emergency Management and Business Continuity/Continuity of Operations* (NFPA 1600) on mitigation:

- The entity shall develop and implement a mitigation strategy that includes measures to be taken to limit or control the consequences, extent, or severity of an incident that cannot be prevented.
- The mitigation strategy shall be based on the results of hazard identification and risk assessment, an analysis of impacts, program constraints, operational experience, and cost–benefit analysis.
- The mitigation strategy shall include interim and long-term actions to reduce vulnerabilities.

Stripling noted that legal barriers prevent effective leveraging and information sharing in many communities due to fears of litigation and possible admissions of guilt. He provided the example that the emergency management system is based on the DHS apparatus, which treats all documents as secure documents. Local entities are often uncertain what types of information must be shared based on those legal frameworks without risk of liability. Current guidance emphasizes sharing with health care partners, but lawyers often instruct them not to share, which causes continual conflict.

Anthony Barone, founder and principal advisor, Northern Virginia Emergility, LLC, noted that investigation and intelligence data are rarely used in ICS at the local and state levels. However, he reported that there is an explicit section on ICS in the *National Incident Management System Intelligence/Investigations Function Guidance and Field Operations Guide*, published by FEMA, which describes how and where to integrate research, response, and incident command; it contains explicit mention of where research, epidemiology, and complex biological chemical incidence could fit into ICS.

---

[1] FEMA PS – PREP; NFPA 1600; ISO 22301; ANSI/ASIS Spc.1-2009; TJC/DNV; HHS – sector CIP lead (RIST and THAM).

## LACK OF UNDERSTANDING AND AWARENESS BY THOSE WITH AUTHORITY

Communicating effectively with the people making major decisions about health care and public health preparedness, response, and recovery is a major challenge, according to Alleyne:

> Public health decisions are not necessarily being made by public health professionals or emergency preparedness professionals, which is why there is not a great preponderance of support for developing these critical infrastructures or supporting them at the local level. Decisions are being made by business professionals often focused on the bottom line, who do not value the same rationales for preparedness that health professionals do.

Many policy makers do not understand the difference between public health and health system preparedness, said Hanen, and they require basic education on the entire enterprise, its component parts, agencies' responsibilities, and funding streams. Wolf remarked that the C-suite of the private sector has a vastly different paradigm for communicating, relying heavily on data to explain what needs to be done and why it needs to be done.

## LACK OF INSTITUTIONAL MEMORY AND LONG-TERM CONNECTIVITY

Lien noted that there is a lack of institutional memory within the preparedness arena, partly driven by the annual funding cycle at the local and state levels, as well as a large amount of workforce turnover. She posited that the lack of historical knowledge and institutional relationships is a barrier to effective leveraging and requires rethinking of the same problems time and again. She also noted that practitioners lack resources and time to digest what was learned and translate it into action that can sufficiently tackle all the pieces of these problems.

## RELIANCE ON ACTIVATION OF REDUNDANT SYSTEMS

Hick cautioned that activating continuity of operations and resiliency plans inherently creates risk, because redundant systems are rarely as good as native ones. He stressed the importance of determining with specificity the appropriate thresholds for risk,[2] cost, and delays within the system. For instance, privacy concerns can create delays in sharing life-saving information about a patient (see Box 4-1). Specificity poses a challenge in determining those thresholds, however, because it comes at the price of time, cost, and remediation to the facility. He also cautioned that the right

[2] For example, a once in a 10-, 100-, or 1,000-year event.

**BOX 4-1**
**Controversy Over Functional Needs Registry**

Schmitt raised the issue of the controversy of functional needs registries. He related a story about a disability advocate who opposed a functional needs registry because it would give false hope that help will actually be provided during an incident. Stripling noted that opposition to a functional needs registry is the subject of an ongoing lawsuit in New York City, despite the large data problem with respect to people with functional needs. The current solution has been to build an empty data warehouse, so that in the event of an emergency, there is a procedure that uses existing data-sharing practices to aggregate all existing information about those populations in a single location that can be queried only during the period of that emergency. People who have participated in any of the city's disability programs are queued off with unique identifiers and address information, which satisfies plaintiffs in the lawsuit because they are not being tracked, but they can be queried if needed. Stripling noted that the biggest challenges with data are usually invisible, such as people who are absent from the data. Addressing this challenge requires mapping the gaps to find places where there should not be absences in the data.

SOURCE: Stripling presentation, March 8, 2017.

risk threshold for today is not necessarily the right threshold for tomorrow, given the increasing trend of billion-dollar climate disasters. Determining reasonable thresholds may require outside expertise (such as tiger teams to challenge the infrastructure) that may be costly, but can provide valuable external perspective on the system. He illustrated this point with a flowchart for risk preparedness (see Figure 4-2).

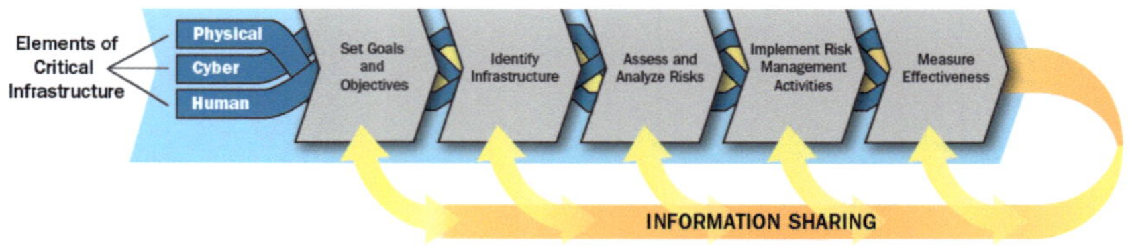


**FIGURE 4-2** Flowchart for risk preparedness.
SOURCES: Hick presentation, March 8, 2017; National Infrastructure Protection Plan, https://www.dhs.gov/sites/default/files/publications/national-infrastructure-protection-plan-2013-508.pdf (accessed August 8, 2017).

Wynia observed that people doing public health work are often so committed and devoted to the mission of helping people that they become "martyrs to the system," absorbing funding cuts and continuing to operate without pushing back. He suggested that from an ethical perspective, there is value to that martyrdom, but from another perspective, it is enabling: "There is a critical intersection between personal devotion and resilience and enabling organizational malfeasance and bad decisions to continue." Runnels described this tension as arising in part from an "us versus them" mentality and suggested that resolving it will require striking a balance between the mission-driven work in public health and a broader system that has different drivers. Hick commented that the public health sector has historically continued to function, in whatever way possible, in the face of significantly scaled-back resources, but the public needs clear messaging to understand the consequences that scaling back entails.

# 5

# Potential Strategies for Strengthening the Nation's Health Security

Our understanding of the health security and disaster landscape has been evolving, Inglesby remarked. It is an opportune time to rethink some strategies for strengthening the nation's health security by building on successful programs and experimenting with new approaches. Although many workshop participants and presenters seemed to agree that there is room to advance, the numerous suggestions for where and how the improvements should be implemented demonstrated that focus, prioritization, and agreement among stakeholders are a necessary first step. By developing and realizing a collective vision, we can advance health security in the United States.

## RETHINKING STRATEGIES

Dodgen called for shifting the conversation away from reacting to the most recent disaster response. He explained that devoting attention to the past is part of why funds are consistently appropriated to singular types of disaster or response strategies rather than system-wide preparedness and resilience. Evolve toward construing preparedness as a general concept, suggested Kurilla, rather than identifying a threat and then focusing on being prepared for that threat. Putting a one-size-fits-all system in place for responding to a wide range of emergencies will not work, he warned. Similarly, David Blazes, senior program officer, Epidemiology and Surveillance, Vaccine Development, Global Health Program, Bill & Melinda Gates Foundation, suggested focusing on preparedness itself as a significant area, rather than as a precursor to response. Often, Blazes noted, critical gaps are not exposed until a threat presents itself: for instance, the poor quality of dengue diagnostics became apparent only after the emergence of the Zika virus.

## DEVELOPING A SHARED AGENDA

Maher called for a clearer distinction between reactive preparedness (the current state) and proactive preparedness, which should be the nation's objective. Stripling called for national distillation of the mission of health care and public health preparedness, response, and recovery in a way that is specific enough that it can be tied to specific data points and can be measured using an agreed-upon set of metrics in the future.

According to Maher, achieving this goal will require establishing a common definition of the problem and the shared dilemma. Even though each group or each perspective brought to the table will work toward that common objective in a different way, Maher emphasized that the different pieces of the puzzle must fit together: "That is the future of public health emergency management. How do we get to the table to break down some of those barriers, recreate the rules, or evolve the rules so that we can do these things quicker and then they'll be more well thought out, more effective, more efficient, and we can do more with less?"

Phillips also recommended establishing a clear, credible mission, with public and congressional support, that details what is required to fulfill the charge to preserve and protect the nation's health security. She also noted that a global partnership is necessary for domestic preparedness. Hick explained that preparing for a range of physical, cyber, and human threats requires setting goals and objectives, identifying the infrastructure that needs protection, carefully assessing and analyzing those risks to that specific area, implementing risk management activities, and then measuring the effectiveness of those interventions to the degree possible.

Marinissen provided ideas for changing one paradigm by framing international assistance and response as a national security issue rather than a selfless humanitarian act. She illustrated with the example of a long-standing cooperative agreement with Panama that provided a small amount of financial support ($100,000 per year). As a direct result of that existing relationship, Panama was willing to provide desperately needed samples to U.S. labs to develop and validate diagnostics during the onset of the Zika virus outbreak. She warned that in the case of a potential emergency requiring diagnostics and protection for all Americans, as well as the rest of the world, CDC is the only entity capable of doing so rapidly and disseminating the information:

> There are going to be many situations, like MERS-CoV or Zika virus, where we are going to need samples or we are going to need countermeasures or supply chain products from other countries. We have to be very strategic. This does not mean that we are going to help 196 WHO-member states and give our money freely without evaluation, without proper metrics, but we need to be very strategic. We need to see what is the benefit for our nation.

Shah suggested leveraging the fact that most Americans support international efforts to improve health in developing countries. Hanfling called for more direct engagement with international partners, by first looking, in particular, at WHO Global Reform and the Global Emergency Workforce, and then promulgating and moving forward a very distinct strategy that brings states, USAID, HHS, and DoD together as domestic partners to work with international partners in clarifying response objectives. Sharon Medcalf, director and assistant professor, Center for Biosecurity, Biopreparedness, and Emerging Infectious Diseases, University of Nebraska Medical Center, also suggested concentrating on international collaboration, such as by conducting joint forums with WHO, Médecins Sans Frontières, and other international organizations, and beginning with a small number of collaborative projects that are low-hanging fruit.

## PROMOTING A CULTURE OF LEARNING AND SHARING

Multiple participants highlighted the need for the field to adopt a culture of learning and sharing, most notably by culling and applying lessons learned from past experiences, particularly during inter-emergency periods. However, Kurilla advised against focusing too heavily on lessons learned and, in effect, "always fighting the last war." Find balance between celebrating successes and learning from every experience, suggested a participant:

> It is deep in our DNA that every outbreak is a chance to find out what is going wrong; every difficult case is a chance to figure out how to do it better next time. That is how we are trained, how we think, and how we improve. We need to have a very firm barrier between that and also telling the story of the successes. We need to learn things from what we do not do well enough. But at the same time, we cannot be shy about telling stories of successes.

Blazes suggested making failure more transparent and learning from it. Stripling suggested creating an easily accessible national database or data warehouse of lessons learned from 10 years of detailed after-action reports and how they have been applied across jurisdictions, which might be housed at the NLM.

Hu-Primmer explained that rapid data collection, rapid aggregation, rapid transformation, and rapid analytics all feed into a "data life cycle" that helps to refine and better understand what additional data need to be collected. A potential focus area for moving forward, therefore, is facilitating rapid bidirectional communication to ensure there are positive optimal outcomes; to improve preparedness, response, and recovery efficacy and effectiveness; and to make sure decision makers have the right information at the right time.

Research should be integrated into ICS if it can be done on a quick-enough feedback loop that it will actually improve the response, according to Stripling. He noted that in the Zika virus response, they attempted to formally integrate research into ICS via an ongoing quality improvement unit tasked with improving response and partnering with research organizations to carry out collaborative studies. This strategy was not fully successful because the timeline required to carry out sound scientific research is longer than the response timeline.

Do not treat paradoxes the same way you treat problems, advised Pavia: problems have solutions that are achievable through creativity and persistence; paradoxes are fundamental problems that cannot be fixed (e.g., people do not appreciate prevention until something bad happens). He warned that devoting too much effort to attacking paradoxes leads to frustration and that fundamental paradoxes should be accepted as a state of being and the focus should be on problems that can be solved (e.g., how to engage more partners rather than getting them to appreciate preparedness in advance). Phillips urged the government to become more creative and innovative in finding solutions to recurring challenges, such as communicating the importance of health security.

## PRACTICE AND REINFORCEMENT

Effective collaboration, trust building, and understanding others' perspectives can only come from practical experience, noted Runnels: "You cannot think your way into a new way of being." Redd concurred, noting that organizations need experience working with other organizations to improve cross-cultural understanding and operational barriers.

Lien reflected that local communities are being asked to fulfill a tremendous amount of preparedness, response, and recovery capabilities, but they are not being provided with the time and resources to focus on building sustainable systems and infrastructure. She suggested that focusing on a smaller number of objectives, rather than many of them, would improve the ability to achieve sustained long-term improvements.

Exercises are a simple way to practice and reinforce new ways of doing business. Employ a more aggressive exercise schedule to boost collaboration and productivity using serious drills with real evaluations, advised Bruce Evans of the National Association of Emergency Medical Technicians. Marinissen proposed using exercises to bring the complex issues of responding to national and global health security threats to those who have access to the resources and the ability to make decisions. She suggested working with HHS/ASPR and DHS to create a series of exercises on the need to invest in pandemic preparedness targeted to the financial sector (both public and private). Danila made a similar suggestion of carrying out exercises and tabletops with federal and state elected officials about the spread of a highly lethal microbe in the United States to demonstrate the importance of maintaining the core public health infrastructure.

Managers and leaders should reward the behaviors they want to see repeated and avoid inadvertently rewarding the wrong behavior, advised Dodgen. At the policy level, he explained that reinforcements include funding and attention to certain populations and issues, and the few incentives currently available may not be for the right things. He suggested rewarding positive behavior such as "above and beyond" collaboration, multijurisdictional exercise, coordination, and innovation.

## BUILDING THE EVIDENCE BASE FOR POLICY AND OPERATIONS

Many attendees highlighted a need to improve the evidence base for preparedness, response, and recovery. Phillips noted a lack of time spent evaluating progress in the field over the previous 15 years and suggested putting in place an evaluation process to strategically assess what works and what does not across broader and more expansive activities, new responsibilities, new organizational structures, and grant programs that have expanded or collapsed.

Goodman suggested promoting the concept of disaster science, which involves both the inter-emergency science agenda and the during-emergency science agenda (e.g., how to collect data during the event to enable a more effective response). He suggested finding ways to further both those agendas and connect their needs to funding by defining and disseminating science gaps and the research agenda. Develop an action plan to use the ever-increasing amounts of data being collected, not just for the response side, but from a science preparedness perspective[1] commented Phillips, who also cautioned against over focusing on infectious disease at the expense of being continually aware of the threat space.

Arnesen remarked that the NLM is home to the NIH Office of Data Sci-

[1] Phillips noted key questions to consider: What data are a common element? What are we learning from that event? How are we turning that immediately back into preparedness and response?

ence, whose new strategic plan focuses heavily on data science and applying the FAIR—findable, accessible, interoperable, and reusable—principle. She explained that the concept of data preparedness (from the Harvard Humanitarian Initiative) connects data, decision making, and response. The aim is to promote the ability of organizations to be ready to responsibly and effectively deploy and manage data collection and analysis tools, techniques, and strategies in a specific operational context before a disaster strikes. Arnesen suggested collaborating with the field of data science, which encompasses open data, data collections, data integration, interoperability, data analysis, translation, knowledge and information management, and dissemination.

Leesa Lin, Harvard University, suggested developing a "rapid science response," a meaningful, rapid assessment that allows evidence to be used quickly to inform response and decision making. Blazes proposed applying the concept of "precision public health" and promoting open, transparent access to data, because "the best public health decisions will require the best data and in many ways, that equates to the most precise data." He suggested that data precision is an equity issue (e.g., precision of determining the risk of transmission of Zika virus in neighborhoods), because everyone deserves to have that level of precision when public health decisions are made. Data precision will require better disease surveillance, better civil registration, better lab diagnostics, and better education.

## ENCOURAGING THE INTEGRATION OF SYSTEMS

Levy called for a paradigm shift toward conceptualizing health care, public health, the business community, and other sectors as parts of a whole that need to be integrated to provide a better environment for the community at large and better care for the community on a day-to-day basis. She recommended considering what can be done in preparedness and emergency response that contributes to providing everyday care, and conversely, what is being done in everyday care that can also translate into being prepared. Blazes noted that the federated database system has its challenges, but it provides opportunities for incorporating innovations within each of the components for better surveillance and response efforts.[2]

At the local level, Redlener emphasized that effective recovery requires centralized infrastructure coordination (which is currently lacking) to manage local assets, state assets, federal assets, nonprofits, insurance companies, and banks. In the best-case version of recovery, he suggested, surviving victims would have a case manager who is aware of all of the various governmental and nongovernmental assets available and would coordinate them

[2] A federated database system is a type of meta-database management system that transparently maps multiple autonomous database systems into a single federated database.

for the survivors. In the worst-case version of recovery, surviving victims must become their own case managers, despite dealing with tremendous emotional stress, and find available assets, access them, and complete their recovery on their own.

Marinissen offered several suggestions for how the United States could integrate with international preparedness and response efforts, including participating in the worldwide implementation of IHR to establish a better understanding of the world's global capacity to respond to emergencies. She pointed to the WHO Health Emergencies Programme as a clear global lead to coordinate emergency response and called for finding ways for the U.S. system to integrate with that structure, as well as developing frameworks to support WHO. Domestic areas of focus highlighted by Marinissen include a better understanding of how the U.S. ICS and National Response Framework align with the WHO health emergency programs.

When deciding who to bring to the table, include those decision makers as well as the stakeholders who can help push efforts forward, suggested Barone, not just people who are already in agreement about what needs to be done. He suggested including C-level and government decision makers, customers, end users, patients, and other people in the community who have no background in preparedness but who will be using these services as the ultimate endpoint. George also suggested broaching questions and challenges that decision makers are currently facing, or anticipate facing in the near future, to a range of people working across sectors. Think outside the box by bringing in people from outside health care and emergency preparedness to brainstorm, suggested Freda Lyon of the Emergency Nurses Association and vice president of WellStar Emergency Services.

Look to sectors outside the federal government who are studying how to engage with communities, suggested Phillips. Aaron Firoved, National Biosurveillance Integration Center, DHS, advised that when convening stakeholders from across sectors, health care information needs to be translated and considered in practical terms and in other sectors' contexts. Dodgen suggested convening people with different needs and engaging them meaningfully, as well as integrating efforts with existing ongoing activities in other systems. For instance, he suggested targeting groups of people who regularly access government-sponsored social services or health care systems such as home visiting, federally qualified health centers, Meals on Wheels, senior programs, and education systems. He suggested that disaster preparedness could integrate with scout badges, American Red Cross, Voluntary Organizations Active in Disaster, emergency department/EMS actions, or HPP coalitions.

At the nexus of the domestic–international interface, Marinissen suggested strengthening both U.S. domestic health security and international health security through multilateral and bilateral partnerships that would include the creation of frameworks parallel to the international community that could be activated and integrated during an emergency response. Hanfling maintained that coalitions and partnerships matter greatly in response efforts, and that this is an opportunity to build on coalitions like the Coalition for Epidemic Preparedness Innovations and better recognize what resources should be invested within communities, across sectors, and across agencies. Finally, he stressed the importance of supporting rather than slashing budgets.

## OPTIMIZING THE EXCHANGE OF INFORMATION

To mitigate the effects of disasters on health care systems, Margolis emphasized that an interoperable, robust, patient-centered electronic health information exchange (HIE) system must enable clinician and patient access to critical information regardless of where they receive care. George noted that key next steps are finding the appropriate technologies and policies for accessing, protecting, and using information from EHRs to facilitate information exchange in a safe and productive way. Hu-Primmer highlighted several of the legal issues that must be resolved, such as data ownership, data use agreements, patient privacy, and cybersecurity. In an increasingly digital world, she explained, electronic data are constantly being uploaded, downloaded, and transmitted wirelessly via many moving pieces feeding into the same gears,[3] which must be in place and well-greased in advance to facilitate centralized coordination. To be useful, she maintained, these data must be sent to a centralized location so they can be aggregated and available to extract, manipulate, and analyze.

Ensuring interoperability of data across disparate systems nationwide is critical, according to Stevens (see Box 5-1). Successful interoperability requires building trust to share data, he explained. Technical advancements are needed to ensure data can broadly be sent, received, found, and used, but stakeholders must also address inconsistencies across data formats, problems around data quality, and a lack of trust that inhibits sharing. Unique patient identifiers are not currently used in the United States, although Stevens maintained that they would solve many problems with human error and input. Stevens suggested that a key strategy moving forward will be finding ways to ensure the interoperability of electronic health data working across disparate systems across the country. The target outcome is a learning health system enabled by nationwide interoperability that supports all stakeholders, especially individuals and providers (see Figure 5-1).

---

[3] Hu-Primmer noted that these pieces include primary care, specialty care, social services, pharmacies, first responders and EMS, EHRs and other health applications, wearables, hospitals, points of dispensation, and public health.

**BOX 5-1**
**Case Study: California's Patient Unified Lookup System for Emergencies**

Stevens described how the IDEA Lab in Action in California began working toward better interoperability by merging EMS, disaster preparedness, and response to make it actionable in the community. The IDEA Lab looked at possible ways to extend the investment that the government has made in EHRs and HIE to improve patient health, respond to disasters, measure outcomes, and save lives. The goal was to connect 43 separate HIEs in California so that providers and emergency responders have a way to access health information across systems. In Southern California, there are 20 million people, but no single point of connectivity. They aimed to make the system end-to-end compatible by using National Incident Management System III standards that are now clinical document architecture compliant (which makes them compliant with hospital EHRs), by transmitting data from electronic patient care reports and ambulances into hospital EHRs, and then by reaching all the different stakeholders by enabling all providers and practices to connect to local HIEs.

This work led to the development of California's statewide Patient Unified Lookup System for Emergencies (PULSE), explained Stevens. The Office of the National Coordinator for Health Information Technology and ASPR were given $50,000 by the HHS IDEA Lab, $40,000 of which funded a local contractor to build a technical architecture to make it possible to request patient information across all 43 HIE organizations in the state.[a] The target population was displaced victims of disasters and all victims experiencing a medical or trauma emergency served by EMS.[b]

In PULSE, Stevens explained, requested patient query demographics include first and last name, gender, and fields for date of birth and Social Security number. The system is activated inside each EHR (using existing log-on credentials) by a state-declared or federally declared emergency. It is up to the user's discretion to select the candidate(s) from the query results that most likely represent the patient needing treatment during an emergency. During development, it became evident that certain information would be most critical to have during a disaster, such as allergy information and medication lists. Critical information is consolidated in a clinical document architecture that can be queried from any participating HIE in California.

[a] Stevens noted that they used the bully pulpit of California EMS agencies to convince entities to cooperate and share data during an emergency.

[b] Stevens noted that the providers and practices involved were paramedics and EMTs, physicians in emergency departments, physicians working in a mobile field hospital or alternate care site, nurses, and pharmacists.

SOURCE: Stevens presentation, March 8, 2017.

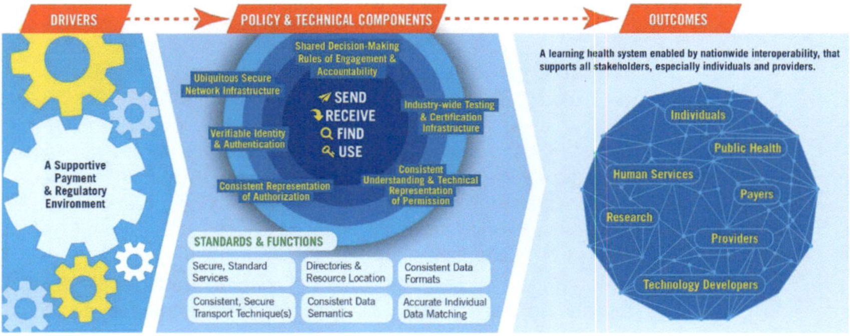


**FIGURE 5-1** Nationwide interoperability of a learning health system.
SOURCES: Stevens presentation, March 8, 2017; from the U.S. Department of Homeland Security.

## SITUATIONAL AWARENESS

Developing a system that creates better health care situational awareness would directly improve decision making, according to Margolis. He recommended promoting greater health care situational awareness as a means of capacity building and system strengthening: "By increasing situational awareness and incentivizing the partners to come together, we can not only improve our preparedness for disasters and public health emergencies, but also make more informed decisions every day." He offered an example from the aviation industry, in which airlines had information about their own safety profile, but were unwilling to share this information due to fears it would be used against them by competitors or the government. To resolve this, the Federal Aviation Administration created and supported the creation of a system known as the Aviation Safety Information Analytic System, a neutral third space to bring everybody together. Through that forum, the airlines identified what information they were willing to share with whom, under what circumstances they were willing to share, and how that information could and could not be used. Most importantly, he noted, this public–private partnership brought the owners of the information together with other interested stakeholders by creating a value proposition that incentivized collaboration. He suggested that a similar system would provide a better understanding of the health care and public health ecosystem (e.g., resources, supply chain, costs, quality, workforce, safety, outcomes, use patterns, planning) during disasters and public health emergencies. Margolis specified that comprehensive situational awareness requires integrating many different data sources, including EHRs, but also other sources of data such as operational data, administrative data, scheduling data, workforce data, inventory management data, and social media information.

## MATCHING DATA TO NEED

Stripling remarked, "We have been hungering for data for centuries, for millennia, but . . . the story is not the data. The story is in the impact. . . . We have to focus on our mission on the territory we have to win. Focus on consequences, why we are doing what we are doing, what those objectives are, what those activities are, how we accomplish it. If we can do that, we will be able to force the data within that framework." He described the New York City health department's approach for focusing on the objective, not the data, in order to avoid going down the "data rabbit hole."

Stripling used the 2015 Legionella outbreak in New York City as an illustration of the importance of defining the mission first, then applying the relevant data. The outbreak was known to be caused by one or more dirty cooling towers in an area around the Bronx borough. The health department began assessments, sampling, and outreach to determine the location of the tainted cooling towers based on epidemiological knowledge. The media questioned the status of the thousands of unregulated cooling towers across the entire city, causing an uproar. Rather than allow the primary mission (i.e., identify the dirty towers) to balloon, the health department stayed focused on the primary objective and the data needed to meet it. After identifying the source of the infection, the mission expanded to include regulating cooling towers.

Map the critical data needed to make decisions, recommended Brinsfield, in order to structure the data to the established mission. She suggested picking out the data pieces that are bridges, measuring them, and then mapping those critical places so that state and local public health agencies are provided with precisely (and only) the data they need to make successful decisions. Runnels suggested incorporating the relevant stakeholders into the development of metrics to ensure that only the critical data are mapped.

## MESSAGING AND MARKETING

Firoved noted that government officials tend to move slowly in crafting the messaging, and if the government is too hesitant to step into that void, someone else will. He recommended that messaging should be early but accurate, and delivered by trusted speakers who have been identified beforehand. For example, he noted that although CDC is one of the gold standards for public trust about health messages, a local health provider or local fire chief is even more effective at the community level.

Dodgen suggested designing messages for people who need to be persuaded to garner funding, attention, and diligence to preparedness: "We tend to design messages for people who are already persuaded." Hick suggested framing messages in ways that can be digested and appreciated in the way that social media are consumed by the public, as well as building local-level trust and using local messengers. Messengers also matter; Laura Holgate, senior fellow, Belfer Center for Science and International Affairs, and visiting scholar, Institute for International Science and Technology Policy, The George Washington University, noted that there is a "ready-made set of civil society communities and private-sector business who all have connection points on the Hill. If we are trying to get the Congress where the American people are, then we need some influencers who are not simply the defenders of federal budgets within the federal government."

Dyjack, Abramson, and Dodgen suggested using storytelling to attract sustained support for and investment in preparedness, response, and resilience. According to Kurilla, public health needs are there and people recognize them, and so creating a narrative about what public health does as a way to make a case to a wider audience and allow them to come to their own conclusions is more effective than trying to convince them of a belief from the public health professional perspective.

## MAKING THE BUSINESS CASE FOR INVESTMENT

Multiple participants suggested the importance of making compelling return on investment (ROI) analyses to catalyze investment in preparedness, response, and recovery. Brinsfield suggested quantifying the cost of inaction and being more transparent with the public about gaps in public health preparedness and the impact on public safety. Develop an ironclad set of priorities and rationale on why health care and public health preparedness investments should not only be maintained but increased, advised Roslyne Schulman, senior associate director, American Hospital Association. Hick stressed the importance of developing convincing arguments in order to demonstrate an ROI, to protect the institution, and to protect the safety of employees and the community. He called for better examples of business impact analysis for health care and compelling case studies for existing health care infrastructure and ROI arguments. Quantify and articulate the potential losses due to a lack of preparedness,[4] suggested Evans, and consider bringing a health economist to the table to assist. Wolf suggested using risk assessment tools and enterprise risk management to make the case for investment. Lin emphasized that evaluation and cost-effectiveness analysis are needed to demonstrate ROI, which will be required to move the public emergency preparedness agenda toward improvements.

---

[4] For example, Evans noted that if a power grid is down for 10 days, what does that loss look like for pharmaceutical sales when a retail pharmacy does not have backup power and cannot scan labels to get medications out?

## FINANCING MECHANISMS

A number of participants suggested solutions for evolving government funding and acquisition rules. At the federal level, Barone proposed finding ways to connect the dots between HHS agencies and to expedite the movement of funds, as well as using contracting and procurement to engage creative minds and innovation from the private sector. As examples of private-sector engagement, he suggested contracting with the private sector to put in place the mechanism of rapid procurement and solicitations. Barone also suggested putting interagency agreements in place to improve the agility of the federal government regarding moving money, as well as adjusting restrictions on how monies can be used during emergencies. Seek out and develop creative funding proposals, suggested Pavia, especially those more closely analogous to insurance, such as an excise tax, that are funded through a constant stream and would allow money to be put forward into a trust fund.

Stripling suggested creating financial guidance to assist local-level public health agencies with the creation of funding packages for federal support and specific assistance for components such as taxes and insurance policies. He additionally suggested producing a financial base plan for diversifying preparedness funding that does not diminish the federal need for grant funding.

Barone drew attention to the overreliance on federal funding and the resulting complacency, arguing that disasters are local, so investment should be local: "Convince local leaders to start investing in local preparedness, or the infrastructure will fail." He noted that federal programs will inevitably change, but reliance on those programs has created local-level expectations that they will continue to receive federal funds in perpetuity. He commented that "businesses and the private sector look at this as business continuity; the government looks at it as continuity of operations; if we don't look at public health in the same way and fail our mission, what's going to happen?"

Consider local-level levers such as surcharges, betterments, or revolving funds to provide resources to support disaster preparedness response and recovery, suggested Runnels. Doug Halley, transportation coordinator, CrossTown Connect, and former director, Acton Public Health Department, noted that in Washington, DC, and other communities with a similar influx of workforce and tourism, it is important to consider every tool possible to understand what the critical need is and what financial mechanisms can be brought to bear. He reported that having partnerships with local businesses has been a useful way to achieve common and overlapping objectives (see Box 5-2).

Lien agreed that there should be more local investment, but warned

**BOX 5-2**
**Case Study: Acton Public Health Department**

Halley noted that fundamentally, emergency preparedness requires both a plan and resources to fund that plan. He offered an example of a local-level solution to the problem of funding. In Acton, Massachusetts, a company discharged contamination into the drinking water supply, shutting down 40 percent of the supply. There was an immediate reactive response to clean up the ground water, coupled with a proactive response to determine if the same contamination might be happening with other companies in the area. This activity led to the creation of a bylaw requiring a permit for facilities to store more than 25 gallons or 25 pounds of hazardous material. Citizens in the community supported the bylaw, but they were not willing to fund it.

Halley's department then created an inspection and permitting scheme that used a revolving account to protect revenue. In addition to inspections and permits, the health department worked with facilities on waste reduction, which further reduced the risk of contamination and allowed them to avoid having to pay for a permit. After 4 years, the department collected enough funds to cover part-time staff, a vehicle, and other inspection costs. After 25 years, the program attained financial stability. Rather than being viewed as a compliance officer, the health department coached facilities on reducing insurance costs and preparing for (and avoiding fines) from state-level inspections. The success of this effort led to cloning the project in other areas. For example, food service is carried out with a revolving account and now generates enough revenue to offset their costs. Halley reflected: "Government is like a glacier; it moves very slowly. You need patience. Perseverance to change the direction of the glacier, you have to have constant force, and a plan in which you know where you're going and how to achieve that."

SOURCE: Halley presentation, March 9, 2017.

that it can be difficult for local communities, coalitions, and health care partnerships to find local businesses willing to contribute, cautioning that there are often a host of assumptions made about how foundations and private-sector businesses are willing to invest. She suggested that communities approach such conversations in more organized ways by helping to define the business case and frame the message to justify and garner investment at the local level and giving it a frame of context so as to justify and present the advantages of investment. Convene private-sector leadership at the national level to discuss priorities and investment preferences, recommended Lien, in order to provide the community-level stakeholders with context and realistic expectations about what they are willing to fund.

# 6

# Future Opportunities

In concluding the workshop, Tom Inglesby reflected on key points made during each of the three panels and four sessions. Presenters and participants discussed, in detail, strategies to address the persistent challenges related to health security, particularly with respect to health care and public health critical infrastructure protection, data collection and use, funding for health security programs, preparedness for global health emergencies, and vulnerable populations and community resilience. Because health security efforts are collaborative and require many levels of national and international governance, discussions reiterated the need for a shared focus on practical, long-term solutions. These strategies are about building a more robust health security infrastructure to minimize the impacts of future disasters that are likely to challenge us.

Inglesby highlighted the importance of leveraging this current transitional period and noted that past and outgoing leaders in health security need to recognize and communicate with new and incoming leadership about the high-level goals and missions of the enterprise (see Box 6-1) and the approaches that have been tried previously to achieve those goals.

Brinsfield urged incoming leadership to maintain focus on the "long game," because even if there are significant changes during a transition, the basic framework and structures in place will endure. Levy advised that transitional periods provide an opportunity for fresh analysis of the utility of existing programs versus new opportunities that may be available. Inglesby concluded by reminding the participants, "We're living in a moment of momentous change, possibly very destructive change, but also possibly change that allows us to reexamine how some of the things that we're doing might be done differently."

**BOX 6-1**
**Advice to the Next Generation Working in Health Security**

During the two keynote panels, participants who held leadership roles in key government agencies in the sphere of health security offered advice to the next generation of leaders:

- Public health students should take into account that the entire field is going to change in the next 20 years and that the current status quo career path may not exist. Maintain your integrity and believe in the mission. (Brinsfield)
- Focus on partnerships, maintain integrity, be part of the team, and establish connections and partnerships. As to the mission itself, support the "boots on the ground" people and remember that public health is actually service. (Levy)
- Become adept at the Federal Acquisition Regulations, because knowing how to move money is useful. (George)
- The corollary in the public health response and preparedness is the "final mile." Regardless of research, knowledge, and degrees, nothing matters if it cannot be implemented at the level at which the emergency is going to happen or before the emergency. You must understand and be connected at the community level of patients and clinicians. (George)
- Always reassess: during an emergency, have multiple points to reassess the situation and to understand changes as the disease emerges and affects risk–benefit or the status of countermeasures. (George)
- Learn to understand the many tribes you may interact with; listen actively and learn effective cross-cultural dialogue. (Vanderwagen)
- Contribute to documenting the evidence base being developed in this arena in a comprehensive and coherent scientific way. (Vanderwagen)
- Continue to learn and recognize the need to do so; engage in situations in which your ideas and beliefs are challenged, and pay more attention to the interfaces your organizations have with others than what your organization is doing. Involve disciplines that are not traditionally part of public health as prominent parts of the operation. (Redd)
- Contribute to bringing an evidence-based scientific paradigm to preparedness and response; bring communities together to build an evidence base across the community, not just internally to the government. (Phillips)
- Turn the lessons learned into lessons applied. (Maher)
- In public health, a pass or defensive move may be as valuable as a goal. (Blazes)

SOURCES: Keynote Panel 1 and Keynote Panel 2, March 8–9, 2017.

# References


Association of State and Territorial Health Officials, NACCHO (National Association of County & City Health Officials), Association of Public Health Laboratories, and Council of State and Territorial Epidemiologists. 2016. Impact of the redirection of public health emergency preparedness (PHEP) funding from state and local health departments to support national Zika response. http://www.naccho.org/uploads/downloadable-resources/Impact-of-the-Redirection-of-PHEP-Funding-to-Support-Zika-Response.pdf (accessed August 8, 2017).

Brunkard, J., G. Namulanda, and R. Ratard. 2008. Hurricane Katrina deaths, Louisiana, 2005. *Disaster Medicine and Public Health Preparedness* 2(4):215–223.

Kaiser Family Foundation. 2016. 2016 Survey of Americans on the U.S. role in global health. http://www.kff.org/global-health-policy/poll-finding/2016-survey-of-americans-on-the-u-s-role-in-global-health (accessed August 10, 2017).

Kappenman, J. 2008. *The future: Solutions or vulnerabilities?* Presentation to the National Research Council's Committee on the Societal and Economic Impacts of Severe Space Weather Events workshop, May 23, Washington, DC.

Kapucu, N. 2005. Interorganizational coordination in dynamic context: Networks in emergency response management. *Connections* 26(2):33–48.

Leider, J. P., B. C. Castucci, C. M. Plepys, C. Blakely, E. Burke, and J. B. Spargue. 2015. Characterizing the growth of the undergraduate public health major: U.S., 1992–2012. *Public Health Reports* 130(1):104–113.

Prina, L. 2017. Public health: What foundations are funding. *Health Affairs* 36(2):376–377.

WHO (World Health Organization). 2011. Disaster risk management for health fact sheets: Child health. http://www.who.int/hac/events/drm_fact_sheet_child_health.pdf?ua=1 (accessed August 10, 2017).

World Bank. 2013. *Strong, safe, and resilient: A strategic policy guide for disaster risk management in East Asia and the Pacific*, edited by A. K. Jha and Z. Stanton-Geddes. Washington, DC: World Bank.

# Appendix A

# Workshop Agenda

## AGENDA

Forum on Medical and Public Health Preparedness for Disasters and Emergencies
Opportunities for the Future of Health Care and Public Health Preparedness, Response, and Recovery: A Workshop
March 8–9, 2017
Location: Room 125, National Academy of Sciences Building
2101 Constitution Avenue, NW, Washington, DC 20418

## WORKSHOP OBJECTIVES

- Examine challenges to medical and public health preparedness, response, and recovery in the context of topics such as global health security, communication and coordination, individual and community health resilience, and critical infrastructure protection.
- Explore the direction of possible future policy actions and innovative approaches necessary to resolving these challenges.
- Discuss possible opportunities for the Forum on Medical and Public Health Preparedness for Disasters and Emergencies and other stakeholders to contribute toward examining and addressing these challenges.

## March 8, 2017

| | |
|---|---|
| 8:30 am (15 min) | **OPENING REMARKS**<br>*Tom Inglesby, Director, JHSPH Center for Health Security* |
| 8:45 am (45 min) | **KEYNOTE PANEL INTERVIEW: THE CURRENT AND FUTURE STATE OF HEALTH CARE AND PUBLIC HEALTH PREPAREDNESS, RESPONSE, AND RECOVERY**<br>***Moderator:*** *Tom Inglesby, Director, JHSPH Center for Health Security*<br><br>***Speakers:***<br><br>*Kathy Brinsfield, Former Assistant Secretary of Health Affairs and Chief Medical Officer, Office of Health Affairs, U.S. Department of Homeland Security*<br><br>*Craig Vanderwagen, Co-Founder and Director, East West Protection, LLC, Former Assistant Secretary for Preparedness and Response, U.S. Department of Health and Human Services*<br><br>*Deborah Levy, Professor and Interim Chair, Epidemiology Department, University of Nebraska Medical Center, College of Public Health, former Lead, Healthcare Preparedness Activity, Division of State and Local Readiness, U.S. Centers for Disease Control and Prevention*<br><br>*Dylan George, Associate Director, B.Next, In-Q-Tel, Former Senior Advisor, Biological Threats Defense, Office of Science and Technology Policy, White House*<br><br>*Jesse L. Goodman, Professor of Medicine, Georgetown University, Former Chief Scientist, U.S. Food and Drug Administration* |
| 9:30 am (30 min) | **AUDIENCE Q/A**<br>***Moderator:*** *Tom Inglesby, Director, JHSPH Center for Health Security* |
| 10:00 am (30 min) | **NETWORKING BREAK** |

10:30 am (90 min) **IGNITE SESSION I: PROTECTING HEALTH CARE AND PUBLIC HEALTH SECTOR CRITICAL INFRASTRUCTURE**

***Moderator:*** *John Osborn, Operations Administrator, Department of Practice Administration, Mayo Clinic*

**What is the existing construct for health care and public health sector critical infrastructure protection and what are the associated challenges?**

***Speaker:*** *Laura Wolf, Chief, Critical Infrastructure Protection Branch, U.S. Department of Health and Human Services*

**How might we better assess the strengths and weaknesses of our health care and public health sector critical infrastructure?**

***Speaker:*** *John Hick, Medical Director, Emergency Preparedness, Hennepin County Medical Center*

**How can the health care and public health sector better collect, validate, and disseminate data on risk and threat information during emergencies?**

***Speakers:***

*Aaron Firoved, National Biosurveillance Integration Center, U.S. Department of Homeland Security*

*Margaret L. Brandeau, Professor of Management Science and Engineering and Medicine, Stanford University*

*Dave Dyjack, Executive Director, National Environmental Health Association*

**FACILITATED SPEAKER AND AUDIENCE DISCUSSION**
***Facilitator:*** *Laura Runnels, LAR Consulting*

12:00 pm (30 min) WORKING LUNCH

12:30 pm (90 min) **IGNITE SESSION II: EMERGING TECHNOLOGY AND RESEARCH/DEVELOPMENT**
***Moderator:*** *Tom Inglesby, Director, JHSPH Center for Health Security*

**How could advances in research and technology impact health care and public health preparedness, response, and recovery?**

***Speaker:*** *Irwin Redlener, Clinical Professor, Health Policy and Management and Pediatrics, Columbia University*

**What are benefits, challenges, and areas of opportunity associated with the use and collection of electronic health data during emergency response?**

***Speakers:***

*Electronic Data – Jean Hu-Primmer, Senior Advisor for CBRN and Pandemic Influenza, U.S. Food and Drug Administration*

*Electronic Health Records – Lee Stevens, Director, Office of State Policy, Office of the National Coordinator for Health IT, U.S. Department of Health and Human Services; and Gregg Margolis, Director, Division of Healthcare System Policy, U.S. Department of Health and Human Services*

*Measurement for Recovery and Future Support – Mitch Stripling, Assistant Commissioner, Bureau of Agency Preparedness & Response, New York City Health*

**FACILITATED SPEAKER AND AUDIENCE DISCUSSION**
***Facilitator:*** *Laura Runnels, LAR Consulting*

2:00 pm (30 min) **NETWORKING BREAK**

2:30 pm (90 min) **IGNITE SESSION III: COMMUNICATION, COORDINATION, AND ENGAGEMENT**
***Moderator:*** *Timothy Sellnow, Professor of Strategic Communication, University of Central Florida*

**How could the health care and public health sector better integrate the perspectives and needs of the community into emergency response?**

*Speakers:*

*Dan Dodgen, Director, Division for At-Risk Individuals, Behavioral Health, and Community Resilience, Office of the Assistant Secretary for Preparedness and Response*

*David Abramson, Associate Professor, New York University College of Global Public Health*

**How can the health care and public health sector better communicate, coordinate, and engage with the public, media, and policy makers to protect public health interests and advances?**

***Speaker:*** *David Eisenman, Director, Fielding School of Public Health, University of California, Los Angeles*

**How can the U.S. efforts in international public health disaster and emergency response, research, and recovery be strengthened and who should take the lead?**

*Speakers:*

*Maria Julia Marinissen, Director, Division of International Health Security, Office of Policy and Planning, Office of the Assistant Secretary for Preparedness and Response, U.S. Department of Health and Human Services*

*Dan Hanfling, Contributing Scholar, JHSPH Center for Health Security*

FACILITATED DISCUSSION
***Facilitator:*** *Laura Runnels, LAR Consulting*

4:00 pm **PANEL: CHILDREN'S EXPERIENCE IN DISASTERS AND THE PERSONAL AND STRUCTURAL FACTORS THAT AID OR HINDER THEIR RECOVERY**
***Moderator:*** *Tom Inglesby, Director, JHSPH Center for Health Security*

*Speakers:*

*Lori Peek, Author,* Children of Katrina, *Professor of Sociology and Director, Natural Hazards Center, University of Colorado*

*David Abramson, Associate Professor, New York University College of Global Public Health*

AUDIENCE Q/A

| | |
|---|---|
| 5:00 pm<br>(30 min) | **RECAP AND REVIEW**<br>*Tom Inglesby, Director, JHSPH Center for Health Security* |
| 5:30 pm | **ADJOURN DAY 1** |

**March 9, 2017**

| | |
|---|---|
| 8:30 am<br>(15 min) | **OPENING REMARKS**<br>*Tom Inglesby, Director, JHSPH Center for Health Security* |
| 8:45 am<br>(75 min) | **IGNITE SESSION IV: FINANCING AND SUSTAINABILITY**<br>***Moderator:*** *Emily St. Martin Lord, Executive Director, Healthcare Ready* |

**What are the current challenges for financing health care and public health emergency preparedness and response?**

***Speaker:*** *Laura Hanen, Chief, Government Affairs, National Association of County & City Health Officials*

**What are existing or possible models for sustainably financing for health care and public health preparedness?**

***Speakers:***

*Public Health Emergency Fund – Dara Alpert Lieberman, Senior Government Relations Manager at Trust for America's Health*

*Local Perspective – Doug Halley, Transportation Coordinator, CrossTown Connect, former Director, Acton Public Health Department*

**How can the commitment to the Global Health Security Agenda be sustained?**

***Speakers:***

*Rebecca Katz, Associate Professor of International Health and Co-Director, Center for Global Health Science and Security, Georgetown University Medical Center*

*Umair A. Shah, Executive Director, Harris County Public Health*

**FACILITATED DISCUSSION**
***Facilitator:*** *Laura Runnels, LAR Consulting*

| | |
|---|---|
| 10:00 am<br>(30 min) | **NETWORKING BREAK** |
| 10:30 am<br>(45 min) | **KEYNOTE PANEL INTERVIEW: INSPIRING ADVANCEMENT IN HEALTH CARE AND PUBLIC HEALTH PREPAREDNESS DESPITE CHALLENGES**<br>***Moderator:*** *Tom Inglesby, Director, JHSPH Center for Health Security*<br><br>***Speakers:***<br><br>*Stephen C. Redd, Rear Admiral (USPHS), Director, Office of Public Health Preparedness and Response, Centers for Disease Control and Prevention, U.S. Department of Health and Human Services*<br><br>*Carmen T. Maher, Acting Assistant Commissioner for Counterterrorism Policy, U.S. Food and Drug Administration, U.S. Department of Health and Human Services*<br><br>*David Blazes, Senior Program Officer, Epidemiology and Surveillance, Vaccine Development, Global Health Program, Bill & Melinda Gates Foundation*<br><br>*Michael G Kurilla, Director, Office of BioDefense, Research Resources, and Translational Research, Associate Director for BioDefense Product Development, Division of Microbiology and Infectious Diseases, National Institute of Allergy and Infectious Diseases, National Institutes of Health, U.S. Department of Health and Human Services* |
| 11:15 am<br>(30 min) | **AUDIENCE Q/A**<br>***Moderator:*** *Laura Runnels, LAR Consulting* |
| 11:45 am<br>(15 min) | **CLOSING REMARKS**<br>*Tom Inglesby, Director, JHSPH Center for Health Security* |
| 12:00 pm | **ADJOURN DAY 2** |

# Appendix B

# Statement of Task

An ad hoc committee will organize a 1.5-day public workshop in Washington, DC. Through this workshop, the committee will convene individuals with expertise in medical and public health preparedness, response, and recovery research, public policy, and practice to (1) examine related medical and public health preparedness, response, and recovery challenges; (2) explore new and innovative approaches and opportunities for resolving these challenges; and (3) discuss the direction of possible future policy actions.

Specific topics that may be explored in this workshop include

- **Global health security** (e.g., opportunities for strengthening the U.S. health care and public health systems' capacity to detect, prevent, plan for, respond to, and recover from naturally occurring outbreaks and intentional or accidental releases of dangerous pathogens and agents)
- **Communication and coordination** (e.g., opportunities for improving situational awareness, public–private information sharing, threat intelligence sharing, risk communication, and collaboration among multi-sector disaster response and medical and public health networks)
- **Individual and community health resilience** (e.g., opportunities for enhancing and ensuring the resilience of individuals and communities through disaster risk reduction, sustainable financing, the inclusion of health in post-disaster recovery planning efforts, work

with non-traditional sectors, and exploring special considerations needed to strengthen a community after a mass casualty incident)

- **Critical infrastructure protection** (e.g., opportunities for improving health care and public health sector and interdependent sector vulnerabilities, recognition of consequences of cascading and prolonged failures of infrastructure, threats from chemical, biological, radiological, nuclear, and high yield explosives, and the increasing threat and consequences of cyber-attack)

The committee will develop the agenda for the workshop session, select and invite speakers and discussants, and moderate the discussions. Workshop proceedings will be prepared by a designated rapporteur in accordance with institutional guidelines, based on the presentations and discussions held during the workshop. The proceedings will be subject to appropriate review procedures before release.

# Appendix C

# Biographical Sketches of Workshop Speakers and Moderators

**Thomas V. Inglesby, M.D., M.P.H.** (*Planning Committee Chair*), is the director of the Center for Health Security at the Johns Hopkins Bloomberg School of Public Health, a nongovernmental academic organization dedicated to protecting people's health from the consequences of epidemics and disasters and ensuring that communities are resilient to those challenges. He is a professor of medicine and public health at the University of Pittsburgh. Dr. Inglesby's work is internationally recognized in the fields of public health preparedness, pandemic flu and epidemic planning, and biosecurity. He is the chair of the Board of Scientific Counselors, Office of Public Health Preparedness and Response, U.S. Centers for Disease Control and Prevention (CDC). He is also the chair of the National Advisory Council of the Robert Wood Johnson Foundation's National Health Security Preparedness Index. He was a member of the External Laboratory Safety Workgroup appointed by the CDC Director that examined biosafety practices of CDC, the National Institutes of Health (NIH), and the U.S. Food and Drug Administration. He was a member of the 2016 Working Group assessing U.S. biosecurity on behalf of the President's Council of Advisors on Science and Technology. He has served on committees of the Defense Science Board; the National Academies of Sciences, Engineering, and Medicine; the Institute of Medicine; and in an advisory capacity to NIH, the Biomedical Advanced Research and Development Authority, the U.S. Department of Homeland Security, and the Defense Advanced Research Projects Agency. During the past 17 years, Dr. Inglesby has authored or co-authored more than 100 peer-reviewed articles, reports, and editorials on a range of issues related to health security and preparedness for epidemics and disasters. He is the editor-in-chief of the journal *Health Security*, which he helped to establish 13 years ago as the first peer-reviewed journal in its field. He was a principal editor of the *Journal of the American Medical Association*'s book *Bioterrorism: Guidelines for Medical and Public Health Management*. He has been invited to brief White House officials from the past three presidential administrations on national biosecurity challenges and priorities, and he has delivered congressional testimony on a number of issues related to public health preparedness and biosecurity. He is regularly consulted by major news outlets for his expertise. He is a member of the board of directors of PurThread, a company dedicated to developing antimicrobial textiles. Dr. Inglesby completed his internal medicine and infectious diseases training at the Johns Hopkins University School of Medicine, where he also served as assistant chief of service in 1996–1997. Dr. Inglesby received his M.D. from Columbia University College of Physicians and Surgeons and his B.A. from Georgetown University. He continues to see patients in a weekly infectious disease clinic.

**David M. Abramson, Ph.D., M.P.H.,** is the founding director of New York University's (NYU's) Program on Population Impact, Recovery and Resiliency (PiR2), a faculty member of NYU's College of Global Public Health, and an associate faculty member of the NYU Medical School's Department of Population Health. Prior to joining the NYU faculty in 2014, Dr. Abramson was the deputy director at Columbia University's National Center for Disaster Preparedness at the Earth Institute. Dr. Abramson has led a number of major research studies examining the long-term impacts of disasters on communities and on vulnerable populations, including children. These studies include the longitudinal Gulf Coast Child and Family Health Study, post–Hurricane Katrina, which has recently received funding from the National Institutes of Health (NIH) to look at recovery 10 years after the storm, and the Sandy Child and Family Health Study currently being conducted in partnership with Rutgers University with funding from the New Jersey Department of Health. Dr. Abramson is also the co-investigator of the NIH-funded Women's and Their Children's Health Study, exploring the impact of the *Deepwater Horizon* oil spill on children's long-term health in collaboration with Louisiana State University. Among his research-to-action initiatives, Dr. Abramson is the co-founder and co-director of the SHOREline youth empowerment project with Colorado State University's Dr. Lori Peek, a curricular project-based learning program presently operating in a number of Gulf Coast and New York City high schools. In addition to the disaster recovery work related to Hurricanes Katrina and Sandy and the *Deepwater Horizon* oil spill, Dr. Abramson has studied short-term post-tornado community recovery in Joplin, Missouri, disaster recovery planning in four mid-sized U.S. cities, risk communication strategies, and organizational and attitudinal aspects of disaster preparedness. Dr. Abramson received his Ph.D. in sociomedical sciences from Columbia University, with a specialization in political science, and an M.P.H. from Columbia University as well. Over the past 25 years he has conducted research on HIV/AIDS, public health systems research, and civic engagement policy and practice. Prior to entering the field of public health, Dr. Abramson spent a decade as a national magazine journalist, having worked at or written for such publications as *Rolling Stone*, *Esquire*, and *Outside* magazines, among others.

**David Blazes, M.D., M.P.H.,** joined the Bill & Melinda Gates Foundation in May 2016 after serving as a physician epidemiologist in the U.S. Navy. Among many career highlights, he and his family spent 4 years in Peru where he directed the Emerging Infections Department at Naval Medical Research Unit Six. His work there involved developing disease surveillance systems in resource-limited settings, working with local officials in responding to outbreaks, and characterizing several novel pathogens. After returning to Washington, DC, he directed the U.S. Department of Defense's (DoD's) global disease surveillance efforts and contributed to DoD's global health security work. He served as the chief advisor to the Navy Surgeon General on Infectious Diseases as well as on the National Academies of Sciences, Engineering, and Medicine's Forum on Microbial Threats. His academic work has appeared in *Science*, *Nature*, and *The Lancet*, and he recently edited a textbook on technological considerations in disease surveillance. Dr. Blazes graduated from the U.S. Naval Academy, did his medical training at Johns Hopkins University, and then did his residency and infectious diseases fellowship at the Bethesda Naval Hospital.

**Margaret L. Brandeau, Ph.D.,** is the Coleman F. Fung professor of engineering and professor of medicine (by courtesy) at Stanford University. Her research focuses on the development of applied mathematical and economic models to support health policy decisions. Her recent work has examined HIV and drug abuse prevention and treatment programs, programs to control the spread of hepatitis B virus, and preparedness plans for bioterror response. She currently serves on the Board of Scientific Counselors, Office of Public Health Preparedness and Response, U.S. Centers for Disease Control and Prevention (CDC), as well as the National Academies of Sciences, Engineering, and Medicine's Standing Committee for the Centers for Disease Control and Prevention Division of the Strategic National Stockpile. In 2012–2013 she served on the Board of Scientific Counselors/National Biodefense Science Board Working Group for the Strategic National Stockpile Review 20/20 and served on the Institute of Medicine Committee on Prepositioned Medical Countermeasures in 2011. She has published 2 books and more than 100 peer-reviewed papers and has received numerous awards for her research and teaching. Professor Brandeau earned a B.S. in mathematics and an M.S. in operations research from the Massachusetts Institute of Technology and a Ph.D. in engineering-economic systems from Stanford University.

**Kathryn Brinsfield, M.D., M.P.H.,** served as the assistant secretary of Health Affairs and chief medical officer for the U.S. Department of Homeland Security's (DHS's) Office of Health Affairs (OHA) until January 2017. She began her service with DHS in July 2008 and previously served as the director of the Division of Workforce Health and Medical Support within OHA. Before joining DHS, Dr. Brinsfield worked for various organizations, including Massachusetts Homeland Security Boston Emergency Services (EMS), Boston Metropolitan Medical Response System (MMRS), and the del Valle Emergency Preparedness Training Institute. Dr. Brinsfield left Boston as an associate professor at the Boston University Schools of Medicine and Public Health with 13 years of experience as an attending physician at Boston City Hospital/Boston Medical Center. She graduated with honors from Brown University, received her M.D. from Tufts School of Medicine, and received her M.P.H. from Boston University. She completed her residency in emergency medicine at Cook County Hospital in Chicago and her EMS fellowship at Boston EMS. She worked for Boston EMS as the director of research, training and quality improvements, medical director for special operations, and associate medical director. She chaired the American College of Emergency Physician's Disaster Committee, co-chaired the Massachusetts State Surge Committee, assisted in the creation of the Massachusetts Alternate Standards of Care Committee, and was the commander of the Massachusetts-1 Disaster Medical Assistance Team and a supervisory medical officer for the International Medical and Surgical Response Team, which responded to the September 11, 2001, attacks.

**Daniel Dodgen, Ph.D.,** is the director for At-Risk Individuals, Behavioral Health, and Community Resilience in the Office of the Assistant Secretary for Preparedness and Response at the U.S. Department of Health and Human Services (HHS). His office focuses on ensuring that children, at-risk individuals, behavioral health, and community resilience are integrated into federal public health and medical preparedness and response activities. Before joining HHS, Dr. Dodgen served as the special assistant to the CEO and senior legislative and federal affairs officer at the American Psychological Association (APA) following a fellowship with the U.S. House of Representatives Committee on Education. He has served on multiple federal advisory groups and authored numerous articles and book chapters on emergency preparedness, psychology, and public policy. Dr. Dodgen is a trained American Red Cross disaster mental health worker and was part of the response to the 1992 Los Angeles riots, the 1994 Los Angeles earthquakes, the 1995 Oklahoma City bombings, and the September 11, 2001, Pentagon attack. Following the Pentagon attack, Dr. Dodgen co-founded the Metropolitan Washington Mental Health Community Response Coalition and served as its chairman. He received the American Psychological Association 2005 Early Career Award for Contribution to Psychology in the Public Interest and was elected a fellow of APA in 2012. He is a licensed clinical psychologist in the District of Columbia.

**David T. Dyjack, Dr.P.H., Ms.P.H.,** is the executive director and CEO of the 5,000-member National Environmental Health Association (NEHA), a position he has held since May 2015. He contributes to many national and international advisory committees in public health, covering a broad menu of capacity-building initiatives, including adult continuing professional education, formal academic degrees, emergency preparedness, informatics, and environmental health. Under his leadership, NEHA has established a presence in Washington, DC, in support of efforts to influence national policy. Dr. Dyjack earned a doctorate in public health from the University of Michigan, an Ms.P.H. from the University of Utah, and is a board certified industrial hygienist (CIH).

**David Eisenman, M.D., Ms.H.S.,** is the professor in residence at the David Geffen School of Medicine and the Fielding School of Public Health at the University of California, Los Angeles (UCLA), where he is the director of the Center for Public Health and Disasters. Dr. Eisenman's training is in internal medicine, public health, and health services research. He has been funded by the National Institutes of Health, National Science Foundation, U.S. Centers for Disease Control and Prevention, National Institute of Justice, Office of the Assistant Secretary for Preparedness and Response, U.S. Forest Service, Robert Wood Johnson Foundation, and the U.S. Department of Homeland Security to study community resilience to disasters, climate change, violence and the health effects of disasters and trauma. Recent studies investigated the interactions of social and built-environment predictors of heatwave mortality and morbidity, the mortality associated with wintertime extreme heat in Los Angeles, organizational networks in disasters, behavioral responses to wireless emergency alerts, climate change policy in public health, social cohesion and health, wildfires and mental health, and improving treatment for posttraumatic stress disorder in public safety-net clinics. In 2012, the Los Angeles County Department of Public Health appointed Dr. Eisenman as the preparedness science officer for the Emergency Preparedness and Response Program. In 2015, the U.S. National Institute of Standards and Technology appointed Dr. Eisenman to chair the Social and Economic Resilience Committee of the Community Resilience Planning

Guide. Dr. Eisenman is an associate natural scientist at RAND. He holds a board certification in internal medicine and he cares for patients at the UCLA Medical Center.

**Aaron Firoved, Ph.D.,** serves as the director for the National Biosurveillance Integration Center. In this position, he enables a collaboration of federal partners to integrate information about threats to human, animal, plant, and environmental health from diverse sources to develop a more comprehensive picture of the biological threat landscape and support better response decisions. Dr. Firoved also serves as the senior biodefense advisor to the Assistant Secretary for Health Affairs and the chief medical officer of the U.S. Department of Homeland Security. Prior to joining the Office of Health Affairs in April 2012, Dr. Firoved worked for the U.S. Senate Homeland Security and Governmental Affairs Committee where he was responsible for the Committee's programmatic and budgetary oversight of its biodefense, disaster medical response, and medical countermeasure portfolios. Dr. Firoved conducted postdoctoral research studying anthrax pathology at the National Institutes of Health. He received his Ph.D. in microbiology and immunology through studies of bacterial pathogenesis associated with cystic fibrosis disease from the University of Michigan and his B.S. in microbiology from the University of Washington.

**Dylan George, Ph.D.,** is the associate director of B.Next at In-Q-Tel (IQT), a private, nonprofit strategic investment firm that effectively brings leading edge technological innovation to departments and agencies within the U.S. government through targeted support of venture-backed start-up firms. Within IQT, Dr. George helped define and establish a strategic IQT initiative, B.Next, that aims to identify opportunities and risks in the rapidly advancing fields of biological sciences. For B.Next, Dr. George provides strategic science and technical vision to strengthen the capacity within the United States to counter biological threats, specifically those from infectious disease epidemics, whether natural, accidental, or intentional. Prior to joining IQT, Dr. George served Dr. John Holdren, assistant to the President for Science and Technology and director of the White House Office of Science and Technology Policy (OSTP), as a senior advisor for biological threat defense. Among other responsibilities at OSTP, Dr. George provided technical expertise and interagency coordination supporting the response to the Ebola outbreak in West Africa. From 2013–2014, Dr. George worked in the U.S. Department of Health and Human Services within the Biomedical Advanced Research and Development Authority where he led a team that developed analytical approaches to assess risks from emerging infectious diseases and other mass casualty events. From 2009–2013, Dr. George worked within the U.S. Department of Defense on anticipating and assessing infectious disease risks that would impact mission readiness and force health protection. Dr. George worked at the National Science Foundation (NSF) within the Divisions of Biological Infrastructure and Environmental Biology. While at NSF, Dr. George supported, among other activities, the National Ecological Observatory Network and the Ecology of Infectious Diseases program. Dr. George received his Ph.D. from Colorado State University and focused on quantitative analytical approaches for considering how clinically severe pathogens (e.g., *Yersinia pestis*, rabies) persist within wildlife populations.

**Jesse L. Goodman, M.D., M.P.H.**, is a professor of medicine at Georgetown University, where he directs the Center on Medical Product Access, Safety and Stewardship (COMPASS), which focuses on informing science-based policy to address emerging public health needs. He is an attending physician in infectious diseases at Georgetown University, Washington, DC; Veterans Affairs; and Walter Reed National Military Medical Centers. COMPASS's current activities include being part of the National Capital Region Coalition Against Antimicrobial Resistance and mapping the global spread of carbapenem-resistant enterobacteriaceae. Until February 2014 he was the chief scientist of the U.S. Food and Drug Administration (FDA), a position he assumed in 2009 along with deputy commissioner for science and public health (2009–2012) and was responsible for strategic leadership of FDA's crosscutting scientific and public health efforts. He led the 2009 H1N1 pandemic response and medical countermeasure review for FDA, also serving as a member of the U.S. Department of Health and Human Services senior leadership team and the White House Medical Countermeasure Review Group. From 2003 to 2009 he directed FDA's Center for Biologics Evaluation and Research. As the senior advisor to the Commissioner from 1998–1999, he co-chaired the U.S. Task Force on Antimicrobial Resistance, producing the first Public Health Action Plan to Combat Antimicrobial Resistance. He served on the Decade of Vaccines Research and Development Group and on numerous U.S. Centers for Disease Control and Prevention, National Institutes of Health, U.S. Department of Defense, and World Health Organization (WHO) Advisory Committees, including the WHO Ebola Vaccine Working Group. He currently serves as president and trustee of the U.S. Pharmacopeial Convention (a nonprofit organization that sets standards for medicines and promotes global pharmaceutical quality). He is also on the Scientific Advisory Board of the Coalition on Epidemic Preparedness Innovation and is an independent scientific/medical member of the board of GlaxoSmithKline. Previously, he was the professor and chief of infectious diseases at the University of Minnesota, where his laboratory first isolated the emerging tick borne pathogen *Anaplasma phagocytophilum*. A graduate of Harvard, he received his M.D. from the Albert Einstein

College of Medicine and did residency and fellowship training at the Hospital of the University of Pennsylvania and at University of California, Los Angeles, where he was the chief medical resident. He is board certified in internal medicine, infectious diseases, and oncology and was elected to the American Society for Clinical Investigation and to the National Academy of Medicine.

**Doug Halley** is the director of transportation for CrossTown Connect (CtC) and the Town of Acton. CtC is an innovative public–private partnership Transportation Management Association. CtC provides suburban transportation services that help seniors, people with disabilities, commuters, reverse commuters, and special populations to arrive at their destinations. In 2015 CtC was recognized by the International City/County Managers Association for its achievements. Mr. Halley provides the same services for the Town of Acton, which is one of the members of CtC. For his work in transportation, he has received awards from the 495 MetroWest Partnership, Community Health Network Area 15, and the Local Officials Human Services Council. In 2015 he retired as health director for the Town of Acton after 28 years of service. As health director, he was responsible for a visiting nurse service, a 300,000-gallon per day wastewater treatment plant, and stormwater compliance, as well as all public health programs. As director, he implemented a unique funding system for the programs which relied primarily on fees for services. He was chairman of Massachusetts Preparedness Region 4A for 3 years. He developed and implemented an educational program for the Pine Hawk Archaeological site, which received an award from the Massachusetts Historical Commission. He was recognized by the Massachusetts Health Officers Association with the Michael Saraco award.

**Laura Hanen, M.P.P.,** is the chief of government affairs for the National Association of County & City Health Officials (NACCHO) in Washington, DC. The National Association of County & City Health Departments is the voice of the approximately 2,800 local health departments across the country. These city, county, metropolitan, district, and tribal departments work every day to protect and promote health and well-being for all people in their communities. Ms. Hanen's primary responsibilities are to oversee policy development, federal lobbying, and the Big Cities Health Coalition. Ms. Hanen is also a member of NACCHO's executive management team. Ms. Hanen joined NACCHO in March 2011. Prior to coming to NACCHO, Ms. Hanen was the director of government relations for the National Alliance of State and Territorial AIDS Directors for 11 years, as well as the senior lobbyist for the American Congress of Obstetricians and Gynecologists. Ms. Hanen was a legislative assistant for Congressman Rick Boucher of the Ninth District of Virginia and a legislative assistant in the government relations department of the Biotechnology Innovation Organization. Ms. Hanen received her bachelor's degree from Earlham College in Richmond, Indiana, and a master's degree in public policy from Georgetown University in Washington, DC.

**Dan Hanfling, M.D.** (*Forum Co-Chair*), is a consultant on emergency preparedness, response, and crisis management. He is a contributing scholar at the Johns Hopkins Bloomberg School of Public Health Center for Health Security, clinical professor of emergency medicine at The George Washington University, and adjunct faculty at the George Mason University School of Public Policy. He also serves as a special advisor within the Office of the Assistant Secretary for Preparedness and Response at the U.S. Department of Health and Human Services, focused chiefly on the National Hospital Preparedness Program. Dr. Hanfling spent 18 years as principal consultant to the Inova Health System (Falls Church, Virginia) on matters related to emergency preparedness and response. He continues to practice emergency medicine at Inova Fairfax Regional Trauma Center, and is an operational medical director for a regional helicopter emergency medical services service. He was instrumental in founding one of the nation's first health care coalitions, the Northern Virginia Hospital Alliance, created in October 2002. His areas of expertise include biodefense and mass casualty management, catastrophic disaster response planning with particular emphasis on scarce resource allocation, and the nexus between health care system planning and emergency management. In addition to his hospital and emergency medical service clinical responsibilities, he serves as a medical team manager for the Fairfax County–based Federal Emergency Management Association and U.S. Agency for International Development–sanctioned international urban search and rescue team (Virginia Task Force-1, USA-1), and has responded to catastrophic disaster events across the globe. Dr. Hanfling received his undergraduate degree in political science from Duke University, including a general course at the London School of Economics, and completed his medical degree at Brown University. He completed his internship in internal medicine at Brown University and his emergency medicine training at the combined The George Washington University and Georgetown University residency program. He has been board certified in emergency medicine since 1997.

**John L. Hick, M.D.**, is a faculty emergency physician at Hennepin County Medical Center (HCMC) and an associate professor of emergency medicine at the University of Minnesota. He serves as the associate medical director for Hennepin County emergency medical services and medical director for emergency preparedness at HCMC. He is the medical advisor to the Minneapolis/St. Paul Metropolitan Medical Response System. He also serves the Minnesota Department of Health as the medical director for the Office of Emergency Preparedness and medical director for Hospital Bioterrorism Preparedness. He is the founder and past chair of the Minneapolis/St. Paul Metropolitan Hospital Compact, a 29-hospital mutual aid and planning group active since 2002. He is involved at many levels of planning for surge capacity and adjusted standards of care and traveled to Greece to assist in health care system preparations for the 2004 Summer Olympics as part of a 15-member team from the U.S. Centers for Disease Control and Prevention and the U.S. Department of Health and Human Services. He is a national speaker on hospital preparedness issues and has published numerous papers dealing with hospital preparedness for contaminated casualties, personal protective equipment, and surge capacity.

**Jean Hu-Primmer, M.S.,** is currently the senior advisor for chemical, biological, radiological, or nuclear and pandemic influenza in the U.S. Food and Drug Administration's (FDA's) Office of Counterterrorism and Emerging Threats (OECT). Ms. Hu-Primmer has 20+ years of federal experience within the U.S. Department of Health and Human Services. Her past achievements include the development, implementation and management of OCET's Medical Countermeasures Initiative Regulatory Science Program, which fosters high-priority science and technology projects that facilitate FDA review of medical countermeasures against chemical, biological, radiological, and nuclear and emerging disease threats. Most recently, as a health scientist and project officer in the Influenza Division at the Biomedical Advanced Research and Development Authority (BARDA) within the Office of the Assistant Secretary for Preparedness and Response, Ms. Hu-Primmer served as the program champion for BARDA's universal influenza vaccine program initiative, providing subject-matter expertise in product and clinical development. Ms. Hu-Primmer also led BARDA's continuous manufacturing innovations program, a joint initiative with FDA's Emerging Technologies Team, and worked closely with the Advanced Manufacturing National Program Office to launch the first Commerce-sponsored Manufacturing USA Institute for biopharmaceutical manufacturing. During the early years of her tenure within the federal government, Ms. Hu-Primmer worked as a research scientist both at FDA's Center for Biologics Evaluation and Research and the U.S. Centers for Disease Control and Prevention in the area of influenza vaccine development, immunology, and viral pathogenesis, including research on the highly pathogenic avian influenza A/H5N1. Ms. Hu-Primmer also spent time in her federal career as a regulatory affairs scientist for the National Institutes of Allergy and Infectious Diseases, Division of Microbiology and Infectious Diseases where her responsibility included management of the entire extramural influenza vaccine clinical trials regulatory portfolio for the Division. Ms. Hu-Primmer holds a B.S. in microbiology from Cornell University and an M.S. in molecular and cellular biology from the University of West Florida.

**Rebecca Katz, Ph.D., M.P.H.,** is an associate professor of international health and co-director of the Center for Global Health Science and Security at Georgetown University. Prior to coming to Georgetown, she spent 10 years at The George Washington University as faculty in the Milken Institute School of Public Health. Her research is focused on global health security, public health preparedness, and health diplomacy. Since 2007, much of her work has been on the domestic and global implementation of the International Health Regulations. Since 2004, Dr. Katz has been a consultant to the U.S. Department of State, working on issues related to the Biological Weapons Convention, pandemic influenza, and disease surveillance. Dr. Katz received her undergraduate degree from Swarthmore College, an M.P.H. from Yale University, and a Ph.D. from Princeton University.

**Michael G. Kurilla, M.D., Ph.D.,** is the director of the Office of Biodefense Research Affairs and associate director for Biodefense Product Development for the National Institute of Allergy and Infectious Diseases (NIAID). His primary role is to provide overall institute coordination for the product development of medical countermeasures against bioterror threats. At the University of Virginia, he was an assistant professor of pathology as well as co-director of the Laboratory of Molecular Diagnostics and associate director for clinical microbiology. Dr. Kurilla moved to the private sector working in anti-infective drug development at Dupont Pharmaceuticals, Bristol-Myers Squibb, and Wyeth. He subsequently joined NIAID as a medical officer. In 2005, he was named to his current positions within NIAID. He received his undergraduate degree in chemistry from the California Institute of Technology. He earned his M.D. and Ph.D. from Duke University. Dr. Kurilla took his postgraduate medical training in pathology at the Brigham & Women's Hospital in Boston, Massachusetts, and a postdoctoral fellowship with Dr. Elliott Kieff at the Harvard Medical School as a Life Sciences Research Foundation fellow, followed by a Markey Scholar Award.

**Deborah A. Levy, Ph.D., M.P.H.,** is the professor and interim chair of the Department of Epidemiology in the College of Public Health at the University of Nebraska Medical Center. Dr. Levy is a retired Captain with the U.S. Public Health Service and stationed at the U.S. Centers for Disease Control and Prevention (CDC) for the past 20 years. Most recently, she focused on leading the Healthcare Preparedness Activity, a program she developed beginning in 2003 while in the Division of Healthcare Quality Promotion, which concentrates on all-hazards preparedness and emergency response of the health care system. Her primary interest has been working with communities to assist them with integrating planning of public health, health care, emergency medical services, and emergency management sectors to improve responses to public health emergencies. Dr. Levy's career at CDC began in 1996 as an epidemic intelligence service officer in the Division of Parasitic Diseases, where she studied foodborne diseases such as Cyclosporiasis and oversaw the National Waterborne Diseases Outbreak Surveillance System. Among other roles, Dr. Levy served as acting director of the Division of Strategic National Stockpile. Throughout her time at CDC, Dr. Levy responded to many incidents including severe acute respiratory syndrome, Hurricane Katrina, the 2009 H1N1 influenza pandemic, Middle East respiratory syndrome, Ebola, and Zika. Prior to CDC, Dr. Levy was involved in National Institutes of Health studies in neuro and cancer epidemiology, as well as HIV wasting syndrome. She earned a B.A. in psychology and an M.P.H. in epidemiology from the University of California, Los Angeles, and a Ph.D. in epidemiology from the Johns Hopkins University School of Hygiene and Public Health.

**Dara Alpert Lieberman, M.P.P.,** is the senior government relations manager at Trust for America's Health (TFAH). She works with the director of government relations to advance TFAH's agenda with federal, state, and local governments. At TFAH, Ms. Lieberman leads the organization's advocacy around infectious disease prevention, disease surveillance, and strengthening the nation's public health emergency preparedness and response capabilities. Ms. Lieberman previously served as a legislative representative for the American Counseling Association, where she advocated for mental health access issues. In recent years, Ms. Lieberman has also worked on children's health care access for the Children's Defense Fund and served as a staff member for the Senate Committee on Armed Services. In addition to working directly with policy makers, she has organized grassroots advocacy efforts at the national and state level. She secured an M.P.P. from the Gerald R. Ford School of Public Policy at the University of Michigan. She graduated magna cum laude with a B.A. in public policy studies from Duke University. Ms. Lieberman currently serves on the board of Healthcare Ready, a nonprofit that works to protect patient access to health care in the face of disaster through collaboration with public health and health care.

**Emily Lord, M.P.A.,** is the executive director of Healthcare Ready. She oversees programs that help strengthen health care supply chains through collaboration with public health and private sectors before, during, and after disasters and pandemic outbreaks. As the convener of industry and government, Healthcare Ready safeguards patient health by providing solutions to critical problems, and provides best practices for health care preparedness and response. Ms. Lord has led Healthcare Ready through multiple natural disasters, including Hurricane Sandy. Ms. Lord also serves as the chair of the U.S. Department of Health and Human Services' Critical Infrastructure Protection Program's lab, blood and pharmacy subsector. Ms. Lord holds an M.P.A. from The George Washington University and a B.A. from the University of Wisconsin–Madison.

**Carmen Maher, M.A., Rear Admiral (RADM),** is a nurse officer in the U.S. Public Health Service Commissioned Corps. She is an assistant surgeon general and is currently serving as the acting assistant commissioner for counterterrorism policy and acting director of the Office of Counterterrorism and Emerging Threats (OCET) in the Office of the Chief Scientist, U.S. Food and Drug Administration (FDA). In this capacity, RADM Maher is responsible for providing leadership, coordination, and oversight for FDA's national and global health security, counterterrorism, and emerging threat portfolios. She serves as FDA's point of entry on policy and planning matters concerning counterterrorism and emerging threats, and collaborates across the U.S. government and internationally on actions to advance global health security and U.S. national security. RADM Maher works in collaboration with other U.S. government agencies to define and prioritize requirements for medical countermeasures (MCMs) to respond to public health emergencies, coordinate research for evaluating MCMs, set strategies for deployment and use of MCMs, and facilitate access to MCMs during public health emergencies. RADM Maher also leads FDA's Medical Countermeasures Initiative, a key component of a broad U.S. government program to improve the U.S. capacity to respond quickly and effectively to public health emergencies. RADM Maher has supported MCM and counterterrorism programs at FDA since 2006. From 2002–2006, she served as nurse officer and lead regulatory officer for pre-clinical and early clinical development of infectious disease vaccines and therapeutics at the National Institutes of Health, National Institute of Allergy and Infectious Diseases, Division of Microbiology and Infectious Diseases. RADM Maher began her nursing career in 1993 as an Ensign in the U.S. Navy, assigned to the National Naval Medical Center in Bethesda, Maryland. She has more than 20 years of experience in nursing, regulatory affairs, clinical trials and medical product development, public health, and emergency response. RADM Maher earned an associate's degree and B.S.N. from the University of Puerto Rico. She earned an M.A. in national security and strategic studies with highest distinction from the U.S. Naval War College in Rhode Island and holds a regulatory affairs certification in U.S. health care product regulations.

**Gregg Margolis, Ph.D.,** is the director of the Division of Healthcare Policy for the Office of the Assistant Secretary of Preparedness and Response at the U.S. Department of Health and Human Services. He leads a team of policy experts in formulating, analyzing and implementing policies to build strong, integrated, and resilient health systems that are prepared to respond to and recover from disasters and public health emergencies. Prior to his federal service, Dr. Margolis was the associate director of the National Registry of Emergency Medical Technicians, a nonprofit organization that serves as the national certification agency for emergency medical services professionals. Dr. Margolis has held leadership positions and faculty appointments at The George Washington University, the University of Pittsburgh, and the Center for Emergency Medicine of Western Pennsylvania. In 2009–2010, Dr. Margolis was the first paramedic to be awarded a Robert Wood Johnson Foundation Health Policy Fellowship, where he served in the Office of Senator John D. Rockefeller. Dr. Margolis has more than 20 years of clinical experience in prehospital emergency medicine, including 12 years as a flight paramedic. He is the author of dozens of publications in a wide array of topics in emergency medicine.

**Maria Julia Marinissen, Ph.D.,** is the director of the Division of International Health Security in the Office of Policy and Planning in the Office of the Assistant Secretary for Preparedness and Response (ASPR) in the U.S. Department of Health and Human Services (HHS). She actively participates in White House National Security Council Interagency Policy Committees on global health security and leads HHS and ASPR participation in bilateral and multilateral partnerships focused on strengthening public health emergency preparedness and response programs, policies, and initiatives. She is the U.S. Liaison to the Global Health Security Initiative, a Ministerial-level effort of the G7 countries, Mexico, the European Commission, and the World Health Organization (WHO). She was founder of and chaired the North American Health Security Working Group, which developed North American Plan for Animal and Pandemic Influenza launched by the leaders of the United States, Mexico, and Canada in 2012. Her division serves as an advisor to the HHS Secretary and the ASPR on international preparedness and response matters, coordinates international communication with health authorities and organizations during public health emergencies, and leads the development and implementation of policy frameworks for international assistance with laboratory samples, medical countermeasures, and emergency medical personnel. She co-led the U.S. donation of antivirals and vaccines during the H1N1 (2009) pandemic to WHO and partner countries, and served as a policy coordinator for the HHS Disaster Leadership Group during the Fukushima nuclear power plant event and the Middle East respiratory syndrome-coronavirus outbreak in the Middle

East. Dr. Marinissen supervises the policy management of the U.S. International Health Regulations (IHR) national focal point (NFP), which also monitors IHR implementation in the United States. In 2016, on behalf of the U.S. government, her team led the self-assessment of U.S. capacities and coordination of the U.S. IHR joint external evaluation. Additionally, she oversees capacity building programs for surveillance, early-warning infectious-disease surveillance, laboratory diagnostics, emergency communications, and IHR NFP strengthening in partner countries across the world. In 2006, she joined the ASPR/Biomedical Advanced Research and Development Authority (BARDA) as a science and technology policy fellow sponsored by the American Association for the Advancement of Science, where she developed requirements and contributed to operational planning for development, acquisition, and distribution of medical countermeasures for biological, radiological, and nuclear threats. She has graduated from the Annenberg Leadership Institute in 2009 and Harvard University's National Preparedness Leadership Initiative in 2014. Prior to her career in policy, Dr. Marinissen received the prestigious "Ramon y Cajal" award from the Spanish Ministry of Science in 2004 and led a research group at the Universidad Autonoma de Madrid. She served as a fellow and senior research associate at the National Institutes of Health from 1997 until 2003. She completed her Ph.D. and master's degree in biology at the Universidad Nacional del Sur in Bahia Blanca, Argentina, where she also held teaching positions in general biology and animal physiology. Dr. Marinissen served for 3 years as a U.S. Marine Corps attaché spouse at the U.S. Embassy in Madrid, Spain.

**John Osborn, M.Sc.,** is the operations administrator at the Department of Practice Administration at the Mayo Clinic in Rochester, Minnesota, supporting the Mayo Clinic Care Network and affiliated practices. He is responsible for practice and business development nationwide and provides strategic leadership for e-health products and services. Prior to this assignment, he was the operations manager for general and trauma surgery in the Department of Surgery and administrator of the Mayo Clinic Level 1 and Level 1 Pediatric Trauma Centers. He has been with the Mayo Clinic since 2004. Mr. Osborn also serves as the lead administrator for mass casualty incident planning and response for the Mayo Clinic and is the administrator for business continuity within the affiliated practices. He is currently an assistant professor of Health Care Systems Engineering in the Mayo Clinic College of Medicine. He is an active member of several national organizations, serving on the boards of directors of the Trauma Center Association of America and the Association of Academic Surgical Administrators. He is also a member of the Sector Coordinating Council for health care and public health within the Critical Infrastructure Protection Advisory Committee system and the editorial board of the *American Journal of Disaster*

*Medicine*. Mr. Osborn received a B.A. in political science from the University of Notre Dame in 2001 and his M.S. in decision sciences from the London School of Economics and Political Science in 2004.

**Lori Peek, Ph.D.,** is the director of the Natural Hazards Center and professor in the Department of Sociology at the University of Colorado Boulder. She studies vulnerable populations in disasters and has conducted field investigations in the aftermath of the 9/11 terrorist attacks, Hurricane Katrina, the BP oil spill, the Christchurch earthquakes, the Joplin tornado, Superstorm Sandy, and Hurricane Matthew. Dr. Peek is author of *Behind the Backlash: Muslim Americans After 9/11*, co-editor of *Displaced: Life in the Katrina Diaspora*, and co-author of *Children of Katrina*. *Behind the Backlash* received the Distinguished Book Award from the Midwest Sociological Society and the Best Book Award from the American Sociological Association Section on Altruism, Morality, and Social Solidarity. *Children of Katrina* received the Best Book Award from the American Sociological Association Section on Children and Youth and the Alfred and Betty McClung Best Book Award from the Association for Humanist Sociologists, and was named a finalist for the Colorado Book Awards. Her work has also appeared in a variety of scholarly outlets, including *Disasters*, *Risk Analysis*, *Natural Hazards*, *Natural Hazards Review*, *International Journal of Mass Emergencies and Disasters*, *Child Development*, *Journal of Family Studies*, *Sociological Inquiry*, *Qualitative Research*, and *Children, Youth and Environments*. In 2016, Dr. Peek received an honorable mention for the Leo Goodman Award for Outstanding Contributions to Sociological Methodology from the American Sociological Association Section on Methodology. In 2009, the American Sociological Association Section on Children and Youth honored her with the Early Career Award for Outstanding Scholarship. Dr. Peek is past chair of the American Sociological Association Section on Environment and Technology and is currently the president of the Research Committee on Disasters for the International Sociological Association. She is a board member for the William Averette Anderson Fund, which is dedicated to increasing the number of underrepresented professionals in hazards and disaster research and practice. She is also an appointed member of the National Academies of Sciences, Engineering, and Medicine's Resilient America Roundtable, a member of the oversight committee for the Mitigation Saves study, and a member of the Advisory Committee on Earthquake Hazards Reduction for the National Earthquake Hazards Reduction Program. Dr. Peek earned her Ph.D. in sociology from the University of Colorado Boulder in 2005. She was a research assistant at the Natural Hazards Center from 1999–2005, and a faculty member at Colorado State University from 2005–2016.

**Stephen C. Redd, M.D., Rear Admiral (RADM),** is the director of the Office of Public Health Preparedness and Response (PHPR) at the U.S. Centers for Disease Control and Prevention (CDC). RADM Redd is responsible for all of CDC's PHPR activities. PHPR provides strategic direction, support, and coordination for these activities across CDC as well as with local, state, tribal, national, territorial, and international public health partners. PHPR carries out its mission by emphasizing accountability through performance, progress through public health science, and collaboration through partnerships. RADM Redd received his baccalaureate degree in history in 1979 from Princeton University and his medical degree with honors in 1983 at the Emory University School of Medicine. He trained in medicine at the Johns Hopkins Hospital and completed the 2-year Epidemic Intelligence Service training program at CDC. Prior to joining PHPR, RADM Redd was the director of CDC's Influenza Coordination Unit. As a medical epidemiologist, RADM Redd managed and directed CDC's efforts to prepare and respond to pandemic influenza—a severe influenza pandemic could cause as many as 2 million deaths in the United States and tens of millions of deaths worldwide. As a career officer, RADM Redd served as an officer in the Junior Commissioned Officer Student Training and Extern Program while in medical school and returned to the Public Health Service following medical training. He has more than 29 years of continuous service as a commissioned officer and has undertaken work as diverse as investigating outbreaks of Legionnaires' disease, to devising diagnosis and treatment strategies for malaria in Africa, to leading efforts to eliminate measles from the United States. Before his current assignment as director of the Influenza Coordination Unit, RADM Redd led CDC's efforts to reduce the burden of asthma in the United States in CDC's National Center of Environmental Health. When the H1N1 pandemic struck, RADM Redd served as the incident commander for CDC's 11-month response, which involved more than 3,000 CDC staff and resulted in the vaccination of more than 80 million Americans against the H1N1 influenza virus. RADM Redd is board certified in internal medicine, a fellow of the American College of Physicians, and a member of the Commissioned Officer's Association. RADM Redd has authored more than 120 scientific publications, including original peer-reviewed research, textbook chapters, and editorials. His research has spanned the gamut from evaluating the impact of air pollution regulations on deaths from carbon monoxide poisoning to the clinical diagnosis of malaria and pneumonia. RADM Redd has received numerous public health service awards, including the Distinguished Service Medal and the Meritorious Service Medal, and is a member of the Alpha Omega Alpha medical honor society. He has been nominated three times and once won CDC's annual Shepard Award for outstanding scientific publications at CDC.

**Irwin Redlener, M.D.,** is a recognized national leader in disaster preparedness and the public health ramifications of terrorism and large-scale catastrophic events. He and his team have developed major programs to enhance public health and health system readiness with respect to disasters. He has written and spoken widely on the response to Hurricane Katrina, U.S. readiness for pandemics, and the concerns of children as potential targets of terrorism. Dr. Redlener has also had more than three decades of experience providing health care to medically underserved children in rural and urban communities throughout the United States. As founder and president of the Children's Health Fund, he is a renowned advocate for access to health care for all children. Dr. Redlener served as a principal developer and president of the new Children's Hospital at Montefiore in the Bronx. He has been a formal and informal adviser to the president and various cabinet members since 1993 and over the past few years has been working with key members of the U.S. Congress on disaster preparedness and child health access. In 1993 and 1994, Dr. Redlener served as a special consultant to the National Health Reform Task Force for the Clinton White House. He has taught medical students in rural Honduras and has led or assisted in international disaster relief in Central America and Africa. Dr. Redlener has also created a series of direct medical relief programs and public health initiatives in the Gulf region ravaged by Hurricane Katrina.

**Laura Runnels, M.P.H.,** is a strategist and facilitator with LAR Consulting, a Washington, DC-based consulting firm. She has more than 12 years of experience providing capacity-building assistance, training, and coaching to local, state, and federal clients. She is known for designing and facilitating highly collaborative, efficient, and productive meetings, workshops, and trainings. As a strategist, she guides individuals, organizations, and coalitions through technical and adaptive challenges. Ms. Runnels holds a master's degree from Saint Louis University and completed her undergraduate studies at Yale University.

**Timothy L. Sellnow, Ph.D.,** is a professor of strategic communication at the Nicholson School of Communication at the University of Central Florida. Dr. Sellnow's research focuses on biosecurity, pre-crisis planning, and strategic communication for risk management and mitigation in government, organizational, and health settings. He has conducted funded research for the U.S. Department of Homeland Security, the U.S. Department of Agriculture, the U.S. Centers for Disease Control and Prevention, the U.S. Environmental Protection Agency, and the U.S. Geological Survey. He has also served in an advisory role for the National Academy of Sciences and the World Health Organization. He has published numerous refereed journal articles on risk and crisis communication and has co-authored five books on risk and crisis communication. Dr. Sellnow's most recent book is titled *Narratives of Crisis: Telling Stories of Ruin and Renewal*. Dr. Sellnow is a recipient of the National Communication Association's Gerald M. Phillips award for Distinguished Applied Communication Research.

**Umair A. Shah, M.D., M.P.H.,** was appointed as the Harris County Public Health (HCPH) executive director and local health authority for Harris County, Texas, the third most populous county in the United States, in May 2013. Since 2004, he served as the HCPH deputy director and director of Disease Control and Clinical Prevention. Prior to joining HCPH he provided clinical care as an emergency department physician at the well-respected Michael E. DeBakey Veterans Affairs Medical Center and chief medical officer at the Galveston County Health District. He earned his B.A. in philosophy from Vanderbilt University and his M.D. from the University of Toledo Health Science Center, where he also completed an international health policy internship at the World Health Organization (Geneva). Dr. Shah completed his internal medicine residency, primary care/general medicine fellowship, and his M.P.H. in management at the University of Texas Health Science Center. Dr. Shah has had a long, distinguished career in public service, having served in numerous leadership positions and having responded to a variety of large-scale emergencies. These include Tropical Storm Allison; Hurricanes Katrina, Rita, and Ike; earthquakes in Kashmir and Haiti; and novel H1N1, Ebola, and Zika outbreaks. Though he is sought nationally for his expertise, Dr. Shah remains actively engaged in both local patient care and academic teaching.

**Lee Stevens** serves in the Office of the National Coordinator as the division director for state policy, overseeing the development and dissemination of policies intended to support the electronic exchange of health information. Mr. Stevens has also served as the manager of the health information exchange (HIE) plan development and oversight for the Eastern and Southern regions of the United States, Puerto Rico, and the Virgin Islands, including technical assistance and long-term planning activities related to enabling exchange. Mr. Stevens also serves as the liaison for intergovernmental affairs on issues related to health information technology (HIT) for the Office of the Secretary. Before coming to the U.S. Department of Health and Human Services, Mr. Stevens served as the federal policy director for the Southern Governors' Association where he managed the Gulf Coast HIT Task Force. The Gulf Coast HIT Task Force was created to establish a dialogue on HIE between states impacted by Hurricanes Katrina and Rita. Mr. Stevens has also served as the Washington, DC-based health and human services advisor for North Carolina Governor Jim Hunt and previously as a senior legislative assistant on health issues for former U.S. Congressman Charlie Rose.

**Mitch Stripling, M.P.A.,** oversees agency preparedness efforts at the New York City (NYC) Department of Health and Mental Hygiene, including units for planning, training and exercise operations, and evaluations. He coordinated citywide planning for the 2009 H1N1 pandemic and served as a planning section chief at the department for the responses to Hurricanes Irene and Sandy, the Ebola crisis, and the recent outbreaks of Legionella and Zika. His program also manages the city's current effort to mount a massive canvassing effort after future disasters. His unit has developed nationally recognized threat response guides for 21 of the highest risk scenarios that could impact NYC, a data- and consensus-driven risk assessment methodology, a principal scientific advisor model for public health incident command system, and a strategic planning directive model for civilian use. Prior to working in NYC, Mr. Stripling worked for the Florida Department of Health. There, he helped plan and implement the responses to six federally declared disasters, including the 2004 record-breaking hurricane season and Florida's response in southern Mississippi after Hurricane Katrina. During that time, he developed, rostered, and trained environmental health and other public health strike teams, built national training standards in collaboration with the U.S. Centers for Disease Control and Prevention, and focused on making communities more resilient in the face of environmental threats. Before working in public health, he spent several years providing strategic consulting for Fortune 500 companies and government agencies. He began his career working at the United Nations Global Teaching and Learning Project on human rights issues.

**W. Craig Vanderwagen, M.D., Rear Admiral (RADM),** serves as the co-founder and director of East West Protection, LLC. Dr. Vanderwagen served for 28 years as a uniformed officer in the U.S. Public Health Service, retiring with the rank of rear admiral (upper half). He served for 25 years in the Indian Health Service. His last assignment was as the presidentially appointed and Senate confirmed Assistant Secretary for Preparedness and Response (ASPR) at the U.S. Department of Health and Human Services. He also serves as a senior partner with Martin, Blanck and Associates, a professional consulting firm located in Alexandria, Virginia. As the founding ASPR, he implemented new federal legislation that established ASPR as the principal leader for all federal public health and medical response activities to any deliberate or natural disasters in the United States. The legislation established a federal role in the development and utilization of human and other material assets in preparedness and response, as well as systems for deploying and managing these assets in emergency situations. His position also gave him authority and oversight of the federal effort to develop and support a wide range of medical countermeasures (e.g., diagnostics, vaccines, therapeutic drugs, and biologics) against chemical, biologial, radiological, nuclear, and pandemic influenza threats. This oversight responsibility included scientific discovery, product development, licensure, acquisition, and deployment. Dr. Vanderwagen was responsible for the creation of operational plans to address the 15 national threats (including biological threats such as anthrax, smallpox, and plague, as well as threats from nuclear, radiation, and chemical devices, and natural disasters such as hurricanes and earthquakes) supported by appropriate situational awareness, logistics, planning, training, and exercises coordinated through the Secretary's Command Center, an emergency operations center linked to all other federal, state, and local command centers. Dr. Vanderwagen received his M.D. from the Michigan State University College of Human Medicine. He completed his residency in family medicine at the University of New Mexico and is board certified in family practice medicine. He received his bachelor's degree from Calvin College.

**Laura Wolf, Ph.D.,** is currently the chief of the Critical Infrastructure Protection Branch of the U.S. Department of Health and Human Services (HHS). She has held various positions within HHS since 2008, including serving as a senior program analyst, science policy advisor, and science policy analyst. From 2007 to 2008, she served as a congressional science fellow on the Senate Health, Education, Labor & Pensions Committee for the American Society of Microbiology. Dr. Wolf is experienced in hospital and public health preparedness, policy analysis, strategic communications, biotechnology, biochemistry, microbiology, immunology and infectious diseases. She holds a doctorate in biological sciences from the University of California, San Diego, and a B.S. in biology from the Massachusetts Institute of Technology.